LEITH HOSPITAL

1848 – 1988

LEITH HOSPITAL

1848 – 1988

DAVID H. A. BOYD

M.D., F.R.C.P.E.

1990

SCOTTISH ACADEMIC PRESS

EDINBURGH

Published by
Scottish Academic Press Ltd,
139 Leith Walk
Edinburgh EH6 8NS

SBN 7073 0584 5

British Library Cataloguing in Publication Data

Boyd, David H. A.
    Leith Hospital, 1848-1988.
    1. Edinburgh. Leith. Hospitals: Leith Hospital, history
    I. Title
    362.1'1'094134

    ISBN 1-7073-0584-5

Printed in Great Britain by Bell and Bain Ltd., Glasgow

Contents

Illustrations

Foreword

As someone intimately concerned with the business community of Leith for many years and more recently with the organisation of health care in the Edinburgh and Lothian area, I am delighted to write this brief foreword.

David Boyd's book makes fascinating reading, recounting as it does every facet of life in Leith Hospital from its inception in the middle of the 19th century to the present day.

But this story starts much earlier, at a time when cholera, plague and other deadly scourges were all too common. Although inadequate medical facilities were available in Leith, it was the need for a treatment place for fever victims that finally led to the establishment of the hospital.

The book relates the changing role and expansion of the hospital over the years and chronicles the many famous and not so well known doctors who passed through its portals. Among the clinicians who were members of staff and who achieved national and international recognition in their fields were Sir Henry Wade, Sir David Wilkie and Sir Stanley Davidson. Other well known names are Dr Sophia Jex-Blake and Dr Elsie Inglis.

Her need of clinical teaching facilities for her women medical students, following a rebuff from Edinburgh Royal Infirmary, first brought Dr Jex-Blake into contact with Leith Hospital. But an arrangement which got off to a harmonious start, to the benefit of both hospital and student, was sadly to end in bitterness and recrimination and Elsie Inglis' part in this is related.

The achievements and failures, the effects of the war years, the arrival of the NHS and the struggle for survival are all faithfully recorded. But Leith Hospital has survived. The opening of the new out-patient department in February 1989 should be seen as proof of the Health Board's commitment to develop the hospital for its new and valuable role in the life of the local community.

R. B. Weatherstone TD, CA   March 1989
Chairman, Lothian Health Board

Acknowledgements

Firstly, I should like to record my thanks to Mr R. Bruce Weatherstone, Chairman of the Lothian Health Board, for his kindness in the midst of a very busy life, in writing a Foreword to this book.

Many people have made the writing of this history possible by their willingness to help in giving of their time, advice and knowledge. Included amongst these are Dr Christine Johnson and Miss Jeffries of the Medical Archives Centre, Edinburgh, Miss Joan Ferguson and her staff, of the Library of the Royal College of Physicians of Edinburgh, and the staffs, both of the National Library of Scotland and the Central Library, George IV Bridge, Edinburgh. By allowing generous access to personal papers, Dr J. D. A. Gray was of immense help, as were Dr A. E. S. Wood and Dr Prudence Barron. Many others supplied verbal and written information. They include, Dr Haldane Tait, Dr Chalmers Davidson, Mr James A. Ross, Mr J. R. Cameron, Mr I. M. C. McIntyre, Ms. Helen Scott, Dr Neil Davidson, Sir James Fraser, Ms. Sheila Mackay, Mrs Heather Waterston, Mrs Winifred Donaldson, Mr Eric Gilmour, Mr Donald McIntosh, Mr Graham Meikle, Dr George Venters, Ms Elizabeth Wilson and Major A. J. Dickinson.

Information concerning the W.R.V.S. was obtained from Mrs Wilkie, M.B.E., Regional Organiser for Lothian, and comments concerning dietary matters from Miss Fiona Steven. Miss Wendy Ross provided recent information on physiotherapy, Mrs Heggie on electrocardiography, Dr Grieve on radiology, Mrs Davidson and Mrs Scobbie on Samaritan Society affairs and Mrs Downie on voluntary fund raising. Mr K. Crichton and Ms McKellar provided information on administrative matters and Miss Bruce and Sister Forbes on nursing matters.

To William Hopkins and his colleagues thanks are due for the preparation of many of the illustrations. I am grateful to Edinburgh City Libraries for permission to reproduce plate 15 and to the Scotsman Publications Ltd. for plates 11, 18, 22 and 23. I acknowledge permission from the Royal College of Physicians of Edinburgh to reproduce the portrait of Dr D. Berry Hart and permission from the Royal College of Surgeons of Edinburgh to reproduce portraits of Sir Patrick Heron Watson and Sir Henry Wade.

Grateful acknowledgement of financial assistance in the production of this book is made to the Carnegie Trust for the Universities of Scotland, to the Lothian Health Board and the Guthrie Trust of the Scottish Society of the History of Medicine.

The typescript was read and commented on by my wife to whom, in addition, I am grateful for constant encouragement. Dr R. F. Robertson also read the typescript and has been a source of very welcome and generous support.

Finally, a chaotic manuscript was transformed to typescript by Mrs Fiona Clarke whose patient and skilful work it is a pleasure to acknowledge.

CHAPTER I

Introduction

The 19th century was well advanced before Leith had anything we would recognise as adequate hospital provision. Indeed, buildings on the present hospital site were not occupied by patients until 1851 and before then facilities were limited in scope and fragmented in locale. In Scotland in general it was the early part of the 18th century which was characterised by the movement for the erection of hospitals.[1] Leith's larger and wealthier neighbour saw the opening of the Royal Infirmary of Edinburgh in 1729. Glasgow, Dundee and Aberdeen but also Perth, Inverness, Paisley, Greenock and Dumfries had established hospitals by the end of the 18th century or in the first half of the 19th century.[2] This is surprising since by 1861 Leith, with a population of 34,000, was the sixth largest town in Scotland.[3]

Buildings set aside for the care of the sick initially catered in the main for the poor and those unable to be looked after in their own homes. At the beginning of the Christian era they were of ecclesiastical foundation but, gradually, administration passed to municipalities and they became lay institutions. In Scotland hospitia or alms houses, largely concerned with the care of old people, existed long before the Reformation [4] and a medieval hospital with chapel dedicated to St. Nicholas was situated in North Leith.[5]

In early Christian times, healing wells or springs were widely used in Scotland the nearest to Leith being that of St. Triduana at Restalrig. St. Triduana had attracted the unwelcome attentions of a Pictish chief and rather than submit she plucked out her eyes and sent them to him impaled on a thorn. The water from the well had a reputation for healing eye disease and was used into the 20th century even after the well-house was moved.[6]

A leper house was built at Greenside in the parish of Leith in 1520 and in 1575 some buildings in "little London" (near the corner of Bernard Street and Quality Street) were cleared out for the use of convalescents from the plague.[7] The preceptory of St. Anthony was founded in 1430 by Sir Robert Logan, whose motives for doing so were not totally altruistic as he directed that the Logan family were "to be prayit for ilk Sunday till the day of doom" by the beneficiaries of his charity.[8] The monks of the hospital of St. Anthony did what they could to succour the poor, elderly and sick with few resources. With the Reformation, monastic benevolence came to an end but the monks of St. Anthony's were suffered to continue their service to the community. In 1592 the funds of the old hospital were transferred to the kirk session of

1

the parish church on the understanding that they would be used for similar purposes.

From these funds a new hospital, usually designated King James's Hospital, was built in 1614 in the Kirkgate, the name commemorating a charter of King James VI.[9] It was managed by the kirk session and by the masters of the trade incorporations or guilds of the town and supported by subscriptions from the incorporations of Maltmen, Traffickers and Trades of Leith. The Mariners, the wealthiest of the incorporations, had accommodation for their own sick poor at the Mariners Hospital in Trinity House. The inmates of these hospitals were nominated from the poor of the incorporations. King James's Hospital was generally occupied by about twelve old women. The buildings were removed in 1822.[10]

From time to time in Scotland in seasons of great epidemic prevalence accommodation of a kind, usually primitive, was hastily created for patients suffering from infectious diseases and Leith shared this practice. In the 17th century Leith, the main port for sea-going ships, was grievously vulnerable and in the terrible year 1645, 2,451 persons, fully half of the town's population, are said to have died of the plague in six months.[11] Smallpox was another deadly scourge and "fever" was an accepted hazard of life and a common cause of death in the first half of the 19th century. There were in all probability several distinct diseases covered by the same name and it was not until 1865 that deaths from enteric fever were separated off in official reports from those attributed to typhus.[12] Cholera was another justifiably feared disease and in the 1831/1832 epidemic in Scotland there were 20,202 cases and 10,650 deaths.[13]

The beginning of the 19th century, then, saw Leith's facilities for coping with these pestilences and other medical problems woefully inadequate.

The Parent Bodies

It is generally accepted that three bodies formed a nucleus from which the modern Leith Hospital evolved. These were the Humane Society, Leith Dispensary and the Casualty Hospital. An examination of the origins and functions of these institutions is worthwhile since the early functioning of the hospital related largely to the purposes of these bodies and for many years it was possible to discern threads from them running through the hospital administrative and professional structure.

The Humane Society

The origins of this body can be traced to a meeting in a London coffee house in 1774.[14] There, a number of eminent physicians, surgeons and lay citizens, formed the society which was first known by the cumbersome but eminently descriptive title "The Institute for Affording Immediate Relief to Persons Apparently Dead from Drowning!"

From the earliest days it was concerned with spreading knowledge of the then known methods of saving life threatened by drowning and other causes. Information on resuscitation in general was always an important function of the Society. It became the Humane Society in 1776 and the Royal Humane Society in 1787.

Dr William Hawes, one of the founders, consulted among others, the great John Hunter, anatomist, surgeon and investigator and Professor William Cullen of Edinburgh as to appropriate methods of resuscitation. Originally these consisted of (1) warmth, (2) artificial respiration by mouth to mouth inflation with compression of the abdomen and chest, (3) fumigation by the introduction of tobacco smoke into the rectum and colon, (4) rubbing the body, or friction, (5) stimulants, (6) bleeding, and (7) the inducement of vomiting. Several of these were soon discarded and replaced by the use of electricity and respiration apparatus. Dr Charles Kite, in a prize essay in 1788, perhaps gave the first description of a cardiac defibrillator which made use of electricity to restart the heart; in the Society's report of 1789 mention is made of the use of electricity applied to the chest wall in the form of low voltage Galvanism. Kite also designed a pattern of bellows adopted by the Society. By 1809 the Society was able to report that Humane Societies, many of them inspired by the work of the London Society, had been formed in 27 places in Great Britain.

The advantages of the Society came to Edinburgh and Leith in 1788. The *Edinburgh Evening Courant* of June 12th of that year reports that through the application of the Rt. Hon. Lord Balgonie who was Comptroller of the Customs at Edinburgh, the Humane Society at London had offered to the town of Leith apparatus such as was used in London for administering relief to persons apparently drowned. (No doubt this was one of Dr Kite's "bellows"). A meeting of "magistrates, clergy, masters of the incorporations, many respectable citizens, and all the medical gentlemen of Leith", accepted the offer. The doctors in Leith were charged with the task of providing premises to house the apparatus and did so first in the Burgess Close and Bernard Street and later in Broad Wynd. On July 26th a "Notice to the Public" appeared in the press[15] to the effect that the medical gentlemen in Leith, with others, had formed themselves into a society to promote the purposes of the Humane Society in London. This notice went on to appeal for funds and ended by quoting a letter addressed to the Humane Society of Leith from Thomas Young, a teacher in Edinburgh, giving thanks for resuscitating his son after a drowning accident. Thus started the work of what became known as the Edinburgh and Leith Humane Society.

The Dispensary

The development in many parts of the United Kingdom of institutions for the treatment of the sick poor who did not require admission to hospital was seen particularly in the latter part of the 18th century. The first in Edinburgh, the Royal Public Dispensary, was founded in 1776 by Dr Andrew Duncan senior, (1744-1828).[16] He was a remarkable man; Professor of the Institutes of Medicine at Edinburgh, a founder of societies and dining clubs and a force in the establishment of the Royal Edinburgh Asylum for the Insane. For this latter achievement his name is perpetuated in the Andrew Duncan Clinic of the Royal Edinburgh Hospital. The dispensary provided attendance on the sick poor at West Richmond Street and also provided instruction in practice to senior medical students. As the New Town of Edinburgh developed and expanded the need for similar premises in the north of Edinburgh became apparent and the New Town Dispensary was opened in Thistle Street in 1815.[17] Eastwood writes that this event was surrounded by a degree of bitterness.[18] Perhaps the existing dispensary felt threatened by a rival. Particular bones of contention were that, firstly, the new dispensary proposed to give medicines and advice including obstetrical aid to patients in their own homes, if this was required, and, secondly, that office bearers were to be elected by subscribers. The proponent of the New Town Dispensary was Dr John Thomson who later became Professor of Military Surgery at Edinburgh; the most conspicuous opponent was Dr Andrew Duncan!

Leith Dispensary came into being in 1816. When it and the Humane Society combined in 1825, a set of rules and regulations were set out which referred to the "branch at Leith of the Royal Public Dispensary".[19] From the start the practice at Leith followed the example of the New Town Dispensary in seeing patients in their homes although contrary to the implication in Eastwood's article, the Royal Public Dispensary also allowed for visits to patients in their homes "when the circumstances of the case required it".[20] Leith Dispensary functioned from its premises at 17 Broad Wynd (and not far from the Humane Society rooms). These were cramped and rather unsalubrious. There was a combined laboratory and consulting room and the other room contained one bed. It was almost certainly here that the death took place in 1819 of the only known patient in Leith to have his portrait hung in the Scottish National Portrait Gallery. John Sakeouse was an Eskimo and is depicted in his native dress, holding a harpoon. He arrived in Leith as a stowaway on board a vessel and as a Christian intended returning home to convert to this religion, his fellow countrymen. He had also assisted Captain John Ross in his search for the North-West passage. He died, according to the gallery information "of typhoid in Leith Hospital".

The Dispensary and Humane Society Combined

These two bodies, with premises very close to each other and both meeting a medical need, very sensibly amalgamated to form the Leith

Dispensary and Edinburgh and Leith Humane Society. Its supporters did not lack fame, position in society or aristocratic background. In 1832 seven years after its amalgamation its patrons were His Grace the Duke of Buccleuch and the Rt. Hon. Lord Viscount Melville; its presidents were the Lord Provost of Edinburgh and the senior magistrate of Leith. Amongst the vice presidents was no less a figure than Sir Walter Scott. The extraordinary directors included the ministers of Edinburgh and Leith of all denominations and such luminaries as Sir Francis Drummond, Sir John Sinclair and Henry Cockburn the Solicitor General. There was a Board of ordinary directors which included the Masters of Trinity House, the Merchant Company, the Maltmen and the Trades, all of Leith and twelve others and a medical committee of eight, all Leith practitioners with "Mr Andrew Liddle, surgeon assistant and apothecary". There was also a person employed as apparatus and housekeeper.[21]

By the year 1832 the annual report recorded a total of 2,350 sick poor attended. The steady increase in these numbers was attributed to much distress and sickness amongst the working classes "arising chiefly from want of employment". "Many", the report continued, "who were accustomed to pay for medicine and advice were now obliged to resort to this institution." The limitations of the Society are however acknowledged in the comment that in all cases of typhus fever where the consent of the parties could be obtained, patients were removed as soon as possible to Edinburgh Royal Infirmary. Nevertheless an important service was rendered to the people of Leith in the terms of the notice to the public which follows.

"Patients whose cases admit of their leaving home receive advice and medicines at the rooms of the Institution (17 Broad Wynd) on Mondays, Wednesdays and Fridays at 1 p.m. and all those who cannot attend are visited by Mr MacDougall and in cases of urgency by one of the medical committee.
Attendance for dispensing medicines daily at 12 noon and 7 p.m.
Children of the poor are vaccinated daily at 12 noon.
Cases of injury or sudden illness receive attention at all hours of the day and night.
Means for resuscitation of those apparently dead from drowning are constantly kept in readiness."

The number of cases presenting to the Humane Society aspect of the work in 1832 was eleven, ten of which were successfully resuscitated. The methods used are mentioned in a specific case, that of a boy of twelve years who when admitted "had no pulse nor any other symptoms of animation. He was placed in a warm bath, using at the same time inflation of the lungs [probably with bellows] and friction with hair brushes". In a short time respiration was established. The Society had about nine "receiving houses" about the port; resuscitating apparatus was kept at Lochend during the skating season and drags for conveyance of unconscious patients were deposited at various points around the docks and shore.

Receipts for the year 1832 were £192.17/2d. Expenditure involved £73 for medicines, £50 for the apothecary's salary, £26 for the housekeeper's salary and £22 for leeches, trusses and Galvanic batteries (so presumably electrical stimulation was being used in some resuscitations).

In the report for 1835 mention is made of problems arising from the increasing number of injuries presenting to the Society.[22] "Notwithstanding proximity to the Edinburgh Royal Infirmary" it states, "the dispensary is resorted to in all cases of accident so that it has become in some measure a casualty hospital." No fewer than fifty cases, as far as the limited accommodation of the house could afford, were dealt with. This of course anticipated the next step in the provision of hospital facilities in Leith — the establishment of the Casualty Hospital. Before considering this however mention must be made of an intriguing and important milestone in medical practice which took place about this time and involved doctors associated with the Society.

Intravenous Therapy in the Treatment of Cholera

Included in the Medical Committee of Leith Dispensary and Edinburgh and Leith Humane Society were the names of Dr Thomas Latta, Dr Thomas Craigie and Dr Robert Lewins. They, especially Latta, were associated with a very important advance in the treatment of cholera, a disease which smote Edinburgh and Leith as well as other parts of Britain and Europe with epidemic force in 1831-1832. Cholera is a very dramatic disease and in the absence of appropriate treatment has a mortality of about 60 per cent often within a few hours. The fact that 172 cures for cholera appeared in the medical literature in the 19th century is an indication of the inefficacy of most.[23]

In 1831 an Irishman, W. B. O'Shaughnessy, who had graduated MD in Edinburgh in 1829, made astute observations on the chemical and physical abnormalities produced by cholera, particularly with regard to the serious loss of water and salts from the body[24] He communicated these observations to the *Lancet* and it was this stimulus which induced Latta and Craigie to treat patients with intravenous solutions of saline. Latta's first letter, which also appeared in the *Lancet* and was addressed to the Central Board of Health, London, was dated 23rd May 1832. A letter from Dr Lewins adding more information about Latta's patients and mentioning two cases treated by Craigie, was dated May 27th. To Thomas Latta then may be given the honour of first describing this important development but it is clear that all three doctors were closely involved. In October that year Latta wrote again giving details of five patients, the communication being entitled "Saline venous injection in cases of malignant cholera performed while in the vapour bath".[25] The first patient treated was an elderly female in whom he inserted a tube into the basilic vein and injected six pints of normal salts of the blood (Dr Craigie's prescription was —

Muriat sodae   ℨi
Carbon sodae grx
Aqua calida to lb iii
Solv temp 105°F).

She made a dramatic recovery and was left in the charge of the hospital surgeon. Often however the benefits were only temporary as it was not realised that the concentration of the salts was too low and for this and other reasons the treatment was little used until more understanding of salt and water replacement was universal.

It has been assumed by some that since Latta, Craigie and Lewins lived in Leith, had their practices there and were on the medical committee of the Leith Dispensary, that the patients they treated in such an innovative manner were in Leith, possibly at the premises of the Dispensary and Humane Society at 17 Broad Wynd. There is nowhere any clear indiction of this and the only hospital mentioned in the communications to the *Lancet* is the Drummond Street Cholera Hospital, Edinburgh. Further, the warm bath which was kept in readiness at the Humane Society premises, was not the "vapour bath" referred to by Latta. He averred that "the warm water bath . . . though productive of transitory excitement has had its evil consequences and is therefore out of use". Craigie refers to patients placed on a "heated tin (sic) (?thin) mattress".[26]

Dr Haldane Tait in his account of the 1832 epidemic states that four cholera hospitals were opened in Edinburgh by the Board of Health.[27] They were in Drummond Street (the old hall of the Royal College of Surgeons), Queensberry House, on Castle Hill and in Fountainbridge. A similar Board of Health was formed in Leith and "pursued an enlightened policy along very similar lines to those adopted by the Edinburgh Board". No mention is made of a cholera hospital in Leith but it seems highly unlikely that all Leith patients were transported to Edinburgh hospitals and all Leith physicians travelled to Edinburgh to attend to them.

Physicians from the west of Scotland however had no hesitation in identifying the locus of these events. On June 6th, 1832 the *Scotsman* reported an article by Dr Thomas Thomson from Glasgow Cholera Hospital published in the *Annals of Philosophy*. In this he discusses intravenous therapy and states "it was first tried in Leith by Dr Latta".

The evidence is therefore that Leith patients and Leith physicians (with Thomas Latta to the fore) were involved; that some patients were treated in Drummond Street Hospital but that some were treated, possibly in the Dispensary premises at Broad Wynd or in some temporary unidentified cholera hospital. Unfortunately Thomas Aitchison Latta (1790-1833) did not live long to pursue his work. It is a curious coincidence that his death certificate ("pulmonary consumption") was signed by a doctor who also is part of the history of Leith Hospital — Dr J. S. Combe. Latta had spent his professional life as a practitioner in Leith but had earlier, in 1818 and still a medical student, made an adventurous journey to the Artic on a whaling expedition and made observations on icebergs.[28]

The Casualty Hospital

The year of the establishment of the Casualty Hospital was 1837. The nature of manual work in the industries in Leith and in the docks, with the paucity of safety regulations then in force, meant that serious injuries were increasing. Reference has already been made to the resulting pressures on the Dispensary and Humane Society and these bodies were aware, as indeed was the public, of the extremely painful and dangerous journey for a badly injured person when he or she had to be transported to the Royal Infirmary of Edinburgh.

No new body or group of people were involved in the start of the Casualty Hospital; it was simply an extension of the premises and workload of the Dispensary and Humane Society. The *Scotsman* of the 14th January 1837 reported that from the great success attending the two bodies of the institution their rooms were not suitable to the demands made on them. "The directors therefore have fitted up that large house in Quality Street, [now Maritime Street] lately occupied by the billet master, as a Dispensary and Hospital for this institution." Having inspected the premises the reporter praised the central situation, the number and size of apartments and their adaptations. He predicted an increase in the workload of Mr MacDougall "the active surgeon of the establishment" in the ensuing years. In another newspaper report prominence is given to the large financial outlay by the Society in fitting up this house but it recognised that it supplied "in some measure" the want of a Casualty Hospital. The stage was being set for future progress.

The Community in need of a Hospital

What kind of community was Leith in the 1840s when the public conscience about poor health care facilities began to stir? Leith like many other places suffered in the economic depression that followed the Napoleonic war. Unemployment, poverty, poor housing, hunger and squalour were the lot of many citizens but by the 1840s some recovery was taking place perhaps assisted by local political and administrative changes and heightened community awareness and spirit. In 1832 the Parliamentary Reform Bill bestowed on Leith the privilege of sending a member to parliament (with Newhaven, Portobello and Musselburgh) and in the following year the Borough Reform Act conferred on Leith a separate and independent magistracy.[29] The borough corporations flourished in the form of Trinity House, The Traffickers or Merchant Company, The Maltmen and the Incorporated Trades of which there were nine — wrights, coopers, hammermen, tailors, cordoners, fleshers, barbers, baxters and weavers. Manufacturing industry was strong and included ship building, sail-cloth manufacture, rope works, glass works, saw mills, soap and candle works, distilling and brewing. A paint works had been established and sugar refining was taking place. There was even an enterprising company preserving meat and vegetables in air-tight tins for naval stores. The ports activities flourished; in 1844 there were 210 ships belonging to Leith firms and there were 2,272 ship arrivals at the docks, 381 of them being steam ships. A vigorous trade existed with Russia, Hamburg and Scandinavia but also the Mediterranean, America, East and West Indies and China. A customs house erected in 1812 employed 106 officers and revenues handled in 1843 amounted to £569,684. A Leith banking company was in existence with branches of several other banks in the town.

Nor were the spiritual, intellectual and social needs neglected. In addition to North Leith Parish Church, South Leith Parish Church and St. John's and St. Thomas's churches there were four free churches and three chapels. The High School of Leith was established and Dr Bell's School had 700 pupils being taught on the Madras system. There were two public libraries, the Mechanics Institute and the Speculative Society. A new Town Hall had been built and the Royal Exchange Buildings housed assembly rooms, a library and hotel.

The relief of poverty was undertaken according to the precepts of the time; there was the Society for the Relief of the Destitute Sick, the Female School of Industry and the Boy's Charity School. The Kirk sessions of North and South Leith were concerned with poor relief — all of it "outdoor".

This then was the community of about 30,000 people that had for the care of sick and injured, one outdoor dispensary, an organisation for the treatment of the apparently drowned and a cramped and inconvenient Casualty Hospital. The time had surely come for the establishment of a Leith Hospital.

REFERENCES

CHAPTER I

1. Comrie, J. D. (1932). *History of Scottish Medicine.* Vol. 2, p. 449. London: Baillière, Tindall and Cox.
2. Ibid., pp. 449-463.
3. Pryde, G. S. (1962). *New History of Scotland.* Vol. 2, p. 249. London: Thomas Nelson & Sons.
4. Comrie, J. D. Op. cit., Vol. 1. p. 57.
5. Ibid., p. 119.
6. Ibid., p. 45.

7. Board of Directors and Staff. *The Story of Leith Hospital* (1896). Leith. p. 11.

8. Russell, J. (1922). *The Story of Leith.* p. 60. London: Thomas Nelson & Sons.

9. Marshall, J. S. (1978). *Leith's Greatest Charity.* p. 2. Edinburgh: W. T. McDougall & Co.

10. Russell, J. Op. cit. pp. 116-117.

11. Pryde, G. S. Op. cit. p. 87.

12. Ferguson, T. (1949). *The Dawn of Scottish Social Welfare.* p. 116. London: Thomas Nelson & Sons.

13. Ibid. p. 128.

14. Bishop, P. J. (1974). *A Short History of the Royal Humane Society.* pp. 1-6. London.

15. *Edinburgh Evening Courant.* 26.7.1788.

16. Comrie, J. D. Op. cit. Vol. 2. p. 456.

17. Ibid. p. 456.

18. Eastwood, M. (1973). *The New Town Dispensary.* Western News. Edinburgh.

19. Leith Dispensary and Edinburgh and Leith Humane Society (1832). Sixth Annual Report.

20. Royal Public Dispensary (1823). Report of General Annual Meeting.

21. Leith Dispensary and Edinburgh and Leith Humane Society. Op. cit.

22. Leith Dispensary and Edinburgh and Leith Humane Society (1835). Ninth Annual Report.

23. Bushnan, J. S. (1850). *Cholera and its Cures.* pp. 130-145. London: W. S. Orr.

24. Passmore, R. (1986). *Proceedings of the Royal College of Physicians of Edinburgh.* Vol. 16. p. 171.

25. Latta, T. (1832). *Lancet.* Vol. 2. p. 173.

26. Craigie, T. (1832). *Lancet.* Vol. 2. p. 277.

27. Tait, H. P. (1966). *Book of the Old Edinburgh Club.* Vol. 32. p. 32. Edinburgh.

28. Masson, A. H. B. (1972). *Book of the Old Edinburgh Club.* Vol. 33. pp. 143-148.

29. *New Statistical Account of Scotland* (1845). pp. 771-781. Edinburgh.

CHAPTER 2

The First Two Decades, 1851-1870

It is difficult to identify one individual who might be acknowledged as the driving force behind the establishment of Leith Hospital. The catalyst in the matter might be regarded as the generosity of Mr John Stewart of Laverockbank who through his representatives left £1,000 for the purpose of providing a fever hospital for Leith, on condition that the inhabitants of the town raised an equal sum. However at a public meeting held in the Assembly Rooms, Leith, on the 30th November 1846, and chaired by Provost Hutchison, a debt of gratitude was recorded to the Rev. Dr Harper who, it was said, was "mainly instrumental in bringing the affair to its present position". Some praise must also be given to all the medical practitioners of Leith who made the need for such a venture very clear. Indeed it was the Right Honourable Lord Advocate, Lord Murray, who at this public meeting read a statement from the doctors that "the establishment of a fever hospital was imperative". The statement went on to remind the meeting that the mortality of Leith exceeded by 5 per cent that of any district of Edinburgh and that one cause of this was the difficulty and delay in removing patients to Edinburgh Royal Infirmary.[1] Later, at an annual meeting of subscribers in 1851, it was the Rev. Dr Harper who in turn credited Dr J. S. Combe with originating the idea of engrafting a fever hospital on the other charitable institutions and recommending the best method of using the £1,000 left by Mr Stewart.[2] There is little doubt that special credit must also be given to another Leith medical practitioner, Dr John Coldstream, for his advocacy of and support for the hospital.

From the start the expediency of combining the proposed fever hospital with the existing Dispensary, Humane Society and Casualty Hospital was recognised and at the inaugural meeting of 1846 a formal proposal that this combination be called "Leith Infirmary" was made. Some time was then spent in discussing the propriety of using the word 'infirmary'. The somewhat sycophantic argument was that such a course might be seen as attempting to supersede the Royal Infirmary of Edinburgh whereas in reality a hospital in Leith was only intended as being "supplementary to that noble institution"! The agreed designation therefore became "The Leith Hospital". This first public meeting ended with the formation of a committee and the subscription of £115 in the room.[3]

There appeared to be a determination to maintain momentum as the next meeting took place on 2nd December 1846 at which it was agreed to divide Leith into districts and that ladies and gentlemen and

11

"persons of inferior degree" should be appointed as collectors of funds for each district. A sub-committee was also appointed to find a site.[4] By March of the following year (1847) the collectors and others had done their work and a sum of £3,175 was amassed. In May a constitution and governing structure was proposed. At the annual meeting of subscribers held on the 21st December 1848 the several charities involved were formally united under one management.

About this time however the medical members of the committee felt they had to record their regret that so much time had been spent in endeavouring to get a site, a regret that must have steadily increased as by October 1848 sites were still being considered. It is reported that the *Leith Herald* of the day ironically challenged its readers "to find out the site of the long talked-of Leith Hospital" They would have had a considerable task as the committee had looked at nine different sites, namely, (1) A court with buildings in the Timber Bush. (2) Ground at the foot of the Kirkgate occupied by a dairy. (3) Todd's property at the head of Sheriff Brae. (4) A house and ground at Morton's Entry. (5) Soapworks at the head of Sheriff Brae. (6) Property near the foot of St. Andrews Street. (7) Mr Brunton's house. (8) Property at King Street used as a wood store, and (9) A small park in front of it — Huddaways Park.[5]

By March of 1849 the secretary of the committee was able to report that he had concluded an agreement with the trustees of the late Mr Todd for the purchase of property at the head of Sheriff Brae as the site for the hospital at a price of £250.[6] Three months later it was agreed to adopt the plans of Mr Peter Hamilton, architect, and to accept the contract price of £1,878 for the building. On 11th March 1850 the foundation stone was laid and in a cavity was deposited an account of the nature and origin of the building, newspapers of the day and coins.[8] The building that emerged facing on to Mill Lane was a simple two storey structure of 60 feet by 63 feet with a Roman Doric pedimented portico.[7] The upper flat formed the fever hospital and accommodated four wards and a store room; on the ground floor there were two wards for casualties, a ward with baths for resuscitation of the apparently drowned and a laboratory or dispensary. It was not until July 1851 that on the recommendation of the medical officers, the hospital was opened for fever patients but they were initially not to exceed fourteen in number.[9]

The Leith Hospital was therefore in existence and functioning and under the control of a governing body consisting of a president, two vice-presidents and fifteen directors of whom three were town councillors, two were ministers of religion, two were from the medical officers of the town and eight were from the general body of contributors. There was also a patron, the first being Lord Murray, and an appointed secretary and treasurer.[10] The first committee of office bearers (as recorded rather confusingly in the *Edinburgh Almanac* for 1851) is as follows.

Committee, Wm. Stevenson, DD, Convenor, Provost McLaren, Bailies Rogers, Brotchie, Morrison, and Kinghorn, Geo. Berry, Thos. Young, Rob. Mowbray, Jas. Millar, Thos. Williamson, MD, James Harper, DD, Rev. G. D. Cullen, Wm. Moodie, Thos. Paisley, Jas. Marshall, Jas. White, Jas. Hay, D. H. Robertson, A. Snody, Rob. Paterson, MD.
Treasurer, William Alexander.
Secretary, Alex. Mann, solicitor.
Consulting physician, J. S. Combe, MD.
Medical Committee, John Coldstream, MD, Thos. Williamson, MD, Rob. Paterson, MD, W. Gilchrist, MD, W. Finlayson, MD, A. C. Livingston, MD, John Gillespie, MD, Jn. Henderson, MD, J. Struthers, MD.
House Surgeon, John Gillespie.
Apparatus and House Keeper, J. Ross.

Clinical Work in the Early Days

In the year before the opening of the new hospital the Dispensary had dealt with 2,699 patients, the Casualty Hospital had treated 245 patients and the Humane Society seven patients.[11] The first full year of the Leith Hospital saw 2,344 Dispensary patients (1,200 of them in their own homes), 268 casualty patients, 122 fever patients and eight submersions treated. Of the casualty patients twenty-eight were admitted and six died; of the fever patients nineteen died, many of these being severe typhus fever but there were also cases of smallpox and scarlet fever.[12] In the first two decades of the hospital numbers increased gradually but with considerable fluctuation in the numbers of fever patients until in 1869 the annual report of the hospital recorded a total of 241 inpatients and 4,427 outpatients.[13] It is difficult to obtain details of the pattern of disease treated in the early years but there exists a record of a list of patients in the institution at one point submitted to the directors by the medical officers in 1856 and is as follows.[14]

Name	Disease
Elizabeth Grant	Typhus fever
Katharine Watt	Typhus
G. Dudgeon	Fracture of lower third of leg
William Snodgrass	Ulcer, varicose
Ernest Fornegan	Febrile attack
John Taylor	Bubo
R. Lawrie	Ascites
Archibald Bewick	Fracture of femur
Kitty Michan	Phthisis, last stage
Mary Nally	Burn

D. Burns	Compound fracture of lower third of leg
Willie Law	Fracture of tibia and fibula
James Hope	Ulcer of leg
John MacKay	Fractures of both femurs
William Cairney	Burns
John Cairney	Burns

Infectious diseases occurring in epidemic proportions were always a concern of directors and medical staff at this time, cholera being a particularly frightening prospect. At an annual meeting of subscribers a director opined that it would be impossible to convert the hospital into a cholera hospital in an emergency. It was agreed that the best that could be done would be to grant discretionary powers to the directors to admit cases of cholera before adequate accommodation could be made by the local fever board, provided that this could be done without prejudice to the other fever and casualty patients for whom the hospital was intended. The matter was raised again in 1859 by the local parochial boards requesting that the directors set aside part of the hospital for the reception of cholera patients. The directors could not agree to this but accepted that should one or two cases occur among foreign seamen they would not object to receiving them if other adequate accommodation was unavailable at the time. They added the rider that they would expect expenses to be defrayed by the parochial board.[15] Three years later the medical officers were warning the directors that there was insufficient accommodation for smallpox and typhus cases; the directors responded by decreeing that no more smallpox cases were to be admitted in the meantime.[16] In January 1863 the almost inevitable result on an increasingly overworked staff came with the death from typhus of the house surgeon, Dr MacDougall.[17]

In 1864 223 cases of fever were admitted. The vast majority (201) were typhus fever and these, with thirteen cases of typhoid fever, accounted for twenty-one deaths. The remainder consisted of smallpox, scarlatina and erysipelas. Concern with hospital infection was reflected by the construction of glass partitions between the fever and casualty wards and the introduction of water and soil pipes to the upper part of the building.[18] Two years later (1886) cholera returned. The first intimation is recorded in the *Leith Burghs Pilot* of the 7th July. A seaman on board the *SS Vistula* from Stettin was found to have the disease and the Public Health Committee reacted promptly by building a wooden hospital (at the cost of £100) on the West Pier for patients arriving by sea. The old Cholera Hospital in Giles Street (possibly that used by Dr Latta and his colleagues) was taken for cases arising in the town and steps were taken for the disinfection of "that grievous nuisance, the manure heap in Salamander Street!" Leith Hospital was therefore spared the necessity of admitting these cases but the medical officers and practitioners pressed for a "house of refuge" for families of victims, a soup kitchen, and house visits to identify patients.

Clearly, ten years after the opening of the hospital accommodation was becoming inadequate. The directors in 1863 noted that "Gladstone's Hospital" immediately opposite Leith Hospital was unoccupied and could afford room for a Casualty Department. Sir Thomas Gladstone was contacted but declined to sell.[19] In parenthesis, "Gladstone's Female Asylum for Incurables" had been endowed in 1840 by his father Sir John Gladstone "for the support of females labouring under incurable diseases" and had ten inmates. Sir John was also father of William Ewart Gladstone, Queen Victoria's Prime Minister on four occasions, and was born in Leith in 1764 at a spot marked by a plaque at the corner of Great Junction Street and King Street. By 1867 the first extension to the hospital was forced on the directors and two wards of six beds each were erected at the back of the original building to take casualty cases.[20]

Early Staffing Arrangements

To cope with this clinical workload a house surgeon (the first being Dr Charles D. Doig who was appointed in January 1851 and was in post on the opening of the new hospital) was appointed at a salary of £60 per year. Ultimate clinical responsibility was in the hands of the medical officers, all practitioners in Leith whose numbers varied but eventually stabilised at eight. The house surgeon's relationship with them was detailed at the opening of the hospital in a set of "Rules for the Guidance of the Resident Surgeon" as follows.

1. He shall take the general superintendence of the laboratory instruments and apparatus belonging to the Institution and observe that the same are kept in a state of efficiency; any additions, alterations or repairs of the instruments, apparatus or medicines that may be required, to be intimated to the Visiting Committee or their convenor.

2. He shall be in attendance at the hours of 12 O'C. noon and 7 O'C. evening for the purpose of dispensing medicine and giving medical advice to those whose occupations prevent attendance at the usual hour of consultation 1 O'C. p.m.

3. He shall require to be in attendance at the time appointed for the daily visit of the medical officer, to receive directions as to the treatment and of all indoor cases.

4. He shall take the immediate care and superintendence of the patients resident in the House; at the same time that his treatment is in all cases to be subject to the inspection, revision and amendment if need be of the medical officer in attendance.

5. As the Institution is an Hospital and Dispensary jointly it is expected that the House Surgeon be always in attendance at the Hospital except during such periods as are absolutely necessary for the attendance on the cases of outdoor patients.

6. In all cases of severe accident or disease in which immediate aid or direction may be required, the House Surgeon is first in every instance to communicate with the ordinary medical officer and in the event of his absence or engagement he is to use his discretion in requesting the attendance of any other medical officer.

7. In all cases of *sectio cadaverus* [post-mortem examination] or important operation the House Surgeon is expected to intimate the same with any circumstance of interest connected therewith to each and all of the medical officers that they may attend if desirous.

8. The resident Surgeon shall have apartments in the Hospital and must never absent himself from his duties for more than two or three hours, without having obtained the sanction of the attending medical officer and having provided a substitute, except in the case of illness.

9. He shall admit, should there be sufficient accommodation in the Hospital, all cases designated as fever with the accompanying card of admission when the card is signed by any of the medical officers — (the question as to the numbers to be admitted to be at all times determined by the Directors). He is also at liberty to admit any of his own outdoor cases affected with fever.

10. He shall admit any description of case when he has a written acknowledgement from a responsible party that the expenses of maintenance will be defrayed provided there is room in the Hospital and in cases of death that the funeral charges will also be paid.

11. With regard to the outdoor cases the House Surgeon shall notice that in no instance is he to visit such parties as he may have reason to believe not to come within the objects of the Dispensary nor to attend any case of labour.

12. He shall take the general superintendence and have stated periods of visitation on the outdoor patients and will not require to visit parties intimating their cases after 9 O'C. a.m., at all, unless these are cases of urgency (it being understood that the House Surgeon shall give a liberal interpretation to this regulation).

13. In the event of any ordinary medical officer being called to an outdoor Dispensary case at the time under the charge of the House Surgeon and consider it necessary to prescribe, the House Surgeon is to make up the prescription and to visit the patient within 24 hours thereafter as being still under his own charge unless informed to the contrary.

14.   He shall keep the books belonging to the Dispensary, Casualty Hospital and Humane Society separately in such a manner as will show what has been done in each department. He shall also keep a fever hospital record of all cases admitted specifying as correctly as possible the name, age, place of birth, place of residence previous to admission with the form of fever under which the patient labours and also a journal for hospital cases in which the history, treatment, diet and result shall be entered.[21]

The first recorded consulting physician was Dr J. S. Combe who was joined a year later by Dr John Coldstream who had been one of the medical officers. How often they were called upon for clinical advice is uncertain, probably infrequently and essentially these posts were sinecures. They served in this capacity to 1883 and 1863 respectively. In 1859 Professor James Syme was appointed consulting surgeon and held post until his death in 1870. These were eminent men of their day.

James Scarth Combe (1796-1883) was born in Leith and was a distant relative of the better known Andrew Combe of phrenology fame. He became a Fellow of the Royal College of Surgeons of Edinburgh in 1823 but Napoleon's defeat at Waterloo put an end to his ambition of becoming military surgeon. He spent time in India then returned to practice in Leith and Edinburgh.[22] He presented a paper in 1822 to the Medico-Chirurgical Society of Edinburgh on "A case of Anaemia" with post mortem appearances suggesting the condition was primarily one of the digestive system and which was, with little doubt, pernicious anaemia. This preceeded Addison's description by almost thirty years.[23] As mentioned previously he signed Dr Thomas Latta's death certificate.

John Coldstream (1806-1863) was also born in Leith and at an early age evinced an interest in Christianity and missionary societies. His biographer John Hutton Balfour, Professor of Medicine and Botany in the University of Edinburgh, dwells at length on Coldstream's religious development and preoccupation. He was apprenticed to Dr Charles Anderson of Leith. After graduating MD at Edinburgh in 1827 he studied at Paris being particularly interested in all aspects of natural history. In 1831 he was involved in the cholera epidemic in Leith but became so exhausted that he had to spend the winter at Torquay with his sisters. Balfour records that in 1846 he, with others, appealed to the people of Leith for support for a hospital and obtained large donations from Mr A. Cowan; he also states that Coldstream drew up the regulations for the management of the hospital. The Fellowship of the Royal College of Physicians of Edinburgh was awarded to Coldstream in 1845 and in 1855 he was involved with the opening of a home and school for invalid and imbecile children in Gayfield Square. A photograph of Coldstream probably taken in his mid 40s shows an intense, intelligent but compassionate man.[24] [plate 1]

Professor James Syme (1799-1870) was associated with Leith Hospital only in the last decade of his illustrious life. Syme was appointed to the Chair of Clinical Surgery and became a surgeon to the Royal Infirmary of Edinburgh in 1833. He had earlier opened a surgical hospital in Minto House in Chamber Street, a hospital immortalised by Dr John Brown in the story "Rab and his Friends". He was a brilliant surgeon although of an acrimoneous disposition. He became Joseph Lister's father-in-law in 1856. His clinical and teaching duties at the Royal Infirmary and University must have left him little time for involvement at Leith Hospital.[25]

There is little record of nursing staff at this time. In pre-Nightingale times the standards were low; formal training was non-existent and the character of the usually elderly women employed was often disreputable. The wages offered to these women at Leith Hospital in 1851 was 4/6d. per week with an allowance of food from the House.[26] These and any washer-women employed were controlled by a house-keeper and a matron, usually a married couple, the first employed being James Ross and his wife. The initial wage of £24 per annum for the house-keeper was soon increased by £10 per annum because of the amount of work and they also received emoluments in the form of heating and lighting. The house-keeper was also expected to keep in good order the apparatus of the Humane Society activities of the hospital and he continued to be recorded as keeper of apparatus until 1874. Although the term "matron" was used this person did not carry out the duties or hold the status of the modern matron. At a meeting of directors in 1860 it was proposed that "the numbers of nurses should on all occasions be left to the discretion of the acting medical officer who is also empowered to order the engagement or dismissal of any nurse without necessarily consulting the matron, the duties of the matron in this matter being limited to carrying out the orders of the acting medical officer who is the best judge both of the numbers of nurses required and of the qualifications of individual nurses". The minutes go on "Mrs Mitchell [the matron] henceforth should attend to Dr Thomson [the House Surgeon] and do everything that was required in his room!"[27] Surely nothing could illustrate more strongly the difference between the two concepts of matron!

An important step as regards nursing was taken in 1866 when at the instigation of the hospital treasurer, Mrs Jane Brown was sent for training at King's College Hospital, London.[28] She served Leith Hospital and the community of Leith with devotion for twenty-one years within her remit of visiting outdoor patients. She performed the functions of a modern health visitor, district nurse and social worker. She, for example, dressed sores, enforced cleanliness, prepared diets and reported cases of destitution to the Destitute Sick Society. This was at a time when the Nightingale Training School for nurses had been inaugurated at St. Thomas's Hospital in London in 1860 and steps to provide nursing training at Edinburgh Royal Infirmary were taken only shortly after this.

Like all institutions the hospital was not without its controversies or disagreements amongst staff. An early medical contretemps occured in 1858 when a special meeting of directors and medical officers discussed Dr Harper's intention to use homeopathic remedies in the hospital. The other medical officers claimed they could not hold professional intercourse with him and that the consulting physicians if called into consultation, must refuse to meet him. Dr Harper clearly recognised the implacable opposition of his colleagues to his deviation from orthodoxy and he resigned. Perversely he offered himself for reappointment but he was hoist with his own petard and he ceased to be a member of staff.[29]

Financial Problems

As a charitable institution the hospital had financial problems from the start. It was dependent on donations from the well-to-do, subscriptions from individuals, works and churches and later, funds from public bodies. One of the early benefactors of the hospital was Alexander Cowan of Valleyfield, Penicuik, who between 1851 and 1853 donated £2,000 which contributed greatly to the building, furnishing and equiping of the new hospital. In the 1869 annual report the treasurer recorded an annual expenditure of £988 with a deficit of £16 in receipts.

Detailed expenditure included

Wages	House Surgeon — £60
	AssistantHouse Surgeon — £45
	Superintendent and matron — £60
	Nurses and servants — £110
Food	£280
Maintenance	£200
Medicines	£93
Wines and Spirits	£10

Receipts included

Subscriptions and donations	£34
Workmen etc.	£13
Church collections	£75
Interest on debenture	£146
North Leith Poor Board	£50

South Leith Poor Board	£100
Leith Dock Commission	£20
Rents	£36
Charity boxes	£6
Board of Patients	£33
General subscriptions	£455

The building fund account had a balance due to the bank of £114.

Although many individuals of all classes gave generously the directors often expressed regret that church congregations and the wealthy did not give more. In 1853 only £97 was raised from the "mercantile classes" of Leith.[30] Some said that artisans should give more as it was for their benefit that the hospital existed. The effect was however that in the early years the hospital could afford to admit only 13-14 fever patients at a time and patients had therefore still to be sent to the Royal Infirmary of Edinburgh. At the beginning, the North and South Leith parochial boards were charged ninepence per day for paupers who were admitted to hospital. Thereafter annual contributions were negotiated with these Boards of £50 and £100 respectively. There was no doubt however as to the lowly status of paupers in a charitable institution; vacant beds could be occupied by pauper patients "on the distinct understanding, that if the bed should at any time be required for the more special purposes of the hospital, or if their treatment interferes in any way with that of other patients, they must at once be removed".[31] Leith Dock Commission contributed £20 in respect of dock workers injured and treated at Leith Hospital. It is recorded in the *Edinburgh Evening Courant* of 3rd February 1857 that the High Constables of Leith solicited subscriptions totalling £300. Individual acts of generosity sometimes took unusual forms and emanated from unlikely sources. In December 1864 for example two illustrated lectures on "Pompeii" were given for the benefit of Leith Hospital by John Hughes Bennett, Professor of the Institutes of Medicine at Edinburgh University and a very eminent physician of his day.[32] In the same issue of the *Leith Burgh's Pilot* in which the advertisement for these lectures appeared, an advertisement for codliver oil was printed. G. Dickson Moffat's preparation was extolled by Professor Hughes Bennett as "one of the best and most genuine codliver oils which has ever been made!" The mores of medical advertising have changed!

REFERENCES

CHAPTER 2

1.   *The Scotsman*, 2.12.1846.
2.   Ibid., 11.1.1851.
3.   Ibid. 2.12.1846.

4. Leith Hospital Provisional Committee, Minutes 2.12.1846.
5. Leith Hospital Committee, Minutes 11.10.1848.
6. Ibid., 28.3.1849.
7. Ibid., 11.3.1850.
8. Gifford, J., McWilliam, C. & Walker, D. (1984). *The Buildings of Scotland; Edinburgh.* p. 464. Penguin Books.
9. Leith Hospital, Board of Directors, Minutes 24.7.1851.
10. *The Scotsman*, 11.1.1851.
11. Ibid., 11.1.1851.
12. Ibid., 2.2.1853.
13. Leith Hospital, Annual Report 1869.
14. Leith Hospital Board of Directors, Minutes 8.3.1856.
15. Ibid., 11.8.1859.
16. Ibid., 17.12.1862.
17. Ibid., 6.1.1863.
18. *Leith Burgh's Pilot* 11.3.1865.
19. Leith Hospital Board of Directors, Minutes 12.11.1863.
20. *Leith Burgh's Pilot* 9.2.1867.
21. Leith Hospital Board of Directors, Minutes 24.7.1851.
22. *Edinburgh Medical Journal* (1883). Vol. 28. p. 862.
23. J. D. Comrie. Op. cit. p. 492.
24. Balfour, J. H. *Biography of the late John Coldstream* (1865). p. 160. London: James Nesbit.
25. J. D. Comrie. Op. cit. p. 594.
26. Leith Hospital Board of Directors, Minutes 2.9.1851.
27. Ibid., 2.2.1860.
28. Board of Directors and Staff. *The Story of Leith Hospital* (1896). p. 21.
29. Leith Hospital Board of Directors, Minutes 16.1.1858.
30. *The Scotsman*, 2.2.1853.
31. Marshall, J. S. (1978). *Leith's Greatest Charity.* p. 9. Edinburgh.
32. *Leith Burgh's Pilot*, 24.12.1864.

CHAPTER 3

Achievements and Failures. 1871-1890

At the halfway mark of Victoria's reign great wealth was accruing to the United Kingdom, technology was changing many aspects of the individual citizen's life but Leith like many other industrial towns continued to have major health problems particularly related to infectious diseases and to suffer poverty and some appalling housing.

Zymotic Diseases

The work of the hospital was diversifying as well as increasing. In 1872 306 inpatients were treated of which 138 had fevers, 103 were casualties, seven were submersions and there were fifty-eight "others".[1] In 1890 (admitted to an extended and enlarged hospital) there were 974 inpatients categorised as 290 surgical, 389 medical and 295 fever. Outpatient attendances had risen from 4,947 to 8,057 (which did not include 162 vaccinations and 1,705 teeth extracted!); the District Nurse in that year attended 221 patients making 6,328 visits. The average length of residence of inpatients in 1886 was 28 days and the detailed breakdown of disease encountered in these inpatients in that year is given in Table. 1.[2]

That said, infectious diseases (or zymotic diseases as they were often referred to then) posed many clinical, administrative and public health problems. In 1871 Dr Struthers one of the medical officers complained to the directors of overcrowding in the fever wards.[3] Sadly nineteen years later in 1890 Dr J. Allan Gray, a medical officer to the hospital and part-time Medical Officer of Health for Leith, had cause to make a strong attack on the inadequacy of provision for infectious diseases in the hospital.[4] Dr Gray who was to play several roles in relation to the hospital had received the gold medal for his M.D. thesis on "Observations on the medico-legal investigation of opium" and became an F.R.C.P.E. in 1881. As well as his general practice, hospital and public health duties he found time to be involved with the Volunteers and became Brigade Surgeon Colonel. The problem of overcrowding was intensified by the necessity to close wards temporarily and reduce nursing staff because of lack of funds.[5] Moreover the same staff was tending both fever and casualty patients with the almost inevitable result of cross-infection, and the danger to staff continued with as many as six nurses contracting typhus in 1890.[6] Further staff deaths occurred. Dr Taylor, House Officer dying in 1873 and Dr Marion Ritchie, House Officer and Nurse Wildig in 1890.[7]

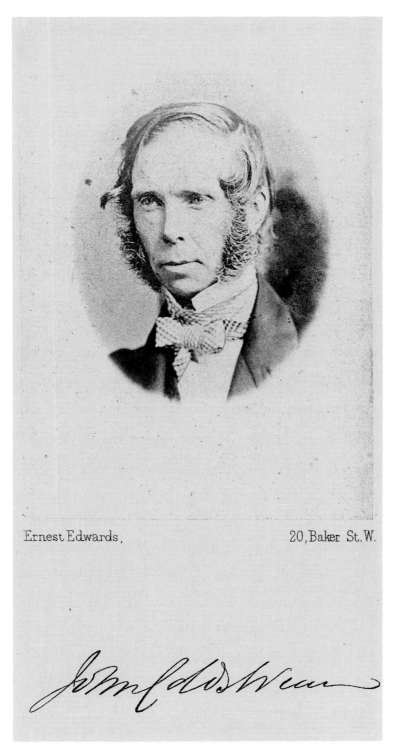

Ernest Edwards,   20, Baker St. W.

PLATE 1. Dr John Coldstream, Consulting Physician, Leith Hospital, 1852-1863

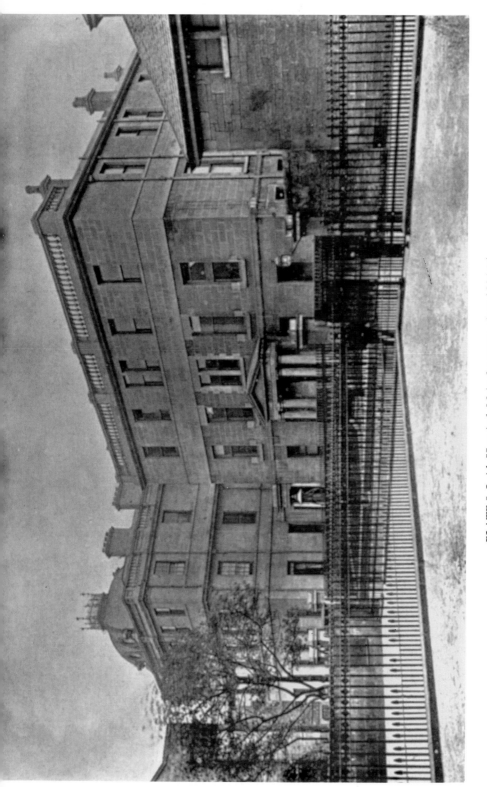

PLATE 2. Leith Hospital. Main frontage, circa 1894-95

It should be remembered that the Public Health (Scotland) Act of 1867 gave powers to local authorities, of which the power to establish hospitals was an important one. The fact that Leith Town Council dragged its feet in this matter was a reason for contentious argument with the directors of the hospital over many years. The council had in fact bought Leith's old Ragged Industrial School in King Street in 1869 when cholera once again threatened.[8] These premises, called the Burgh or King Street Hospital were not opened until 1871 and were unsuitable for the care of fever patients. Nevertheless patients had to be admitted to them during epidemics. The directors of the hospital were resentful that immediately the epidemic was over the premises were closed, that it took some pressure to persuade the council of the presence of another epidemic and in any event it was the directors who had the responsibility of their staffing and administration.

The strife between the directors and the council flared intermittently for over twenty years. In 1881 the directors prepared a memorandum which pointed out the duty of the local authority to provide for cases of infectious disease. It drew attention to the support by councils in other towns for fever hospitals and to the fact that the directors of Leith Hospital as a charitable institution did not have the financial resources to maintain a fever hospital effectively. It went on to remind the council that the hospital received only £100 per annum from the local authority and that the expense of the fever house in any of the years 1870-1880 amounted to about £500.[9] This obviously did not produce the desired effect as in 1888 the secretary to the hospital was writing to the town clerk in terms that virtually amounted to an ultimatum. The letter stated that if the council did not reconsider its position with regard to its contributions "the present agreement should be terminated and that from henceforth they [the directors] will devote the income of the hospital to the dispensary and medical and surgical cases for all of which there is ample field for its expenditure". And there was a Parthian shot — "The town will from the same date require to provide a mortuary of its own".[10] The town clerk replied expressing the somewhat hurt feelings of the council and suggested a meeting which took place on 4th December 1888. This resulted in an agreement that the hospital should undertake care of infectious cases at King Street (cholera excepted) for a capitation payment of £4 from the council.[11] It was not until 1896 however that the East Pilton Fever Hospital (now the Northern General Hospital) was opened by Leith Town Council to meet its obligations.

Hospital Extensions and Finances

In 1870 the directors had also purchased property in King Street and Well Close at a cost of £588 with a view to extending the hospital. They did not however have the financial resources to exploit this at that time. The following year the hospital received a very generous legacy from Mr Thomas Williamson Ramsay of Lixmount of £24,855. This generosity was so well received that new hospital buildings made possible thereby were named the Williamson Ramsay wards[13] and a marble bust of the donor was commissioned, an artifact still in possession of the Lothian Health Board. The buildings by James Simpson, architect, were erected to the north east of the original building at an accepted estimate of £6,818. Although started in 1873 the building was not ready until 1875 (the contractors blamed strikes amongst the labourers!) and provided room for thirty-six more beds as well as Board Room, Lady Superintendent's room and other apartments. It was finally opened on 2nd April 1875 by the Rev. Mr Mitchell.[14] About the same time, alterations were made to the old building to provide more effectively for the dispensary and nurses accommodation. In 1889 to 1890 the 1870's extension was added to by a French mansard roof which provided further ward accommodation, staff quarters and an operating theatre [plate 2]. The capital fund of the hospital received a substantial boost in 1877 when it was suggested by Mr Wishart, a merchant of Leith, that £1500 be added by the expedient of fifteen individuals giving £100 each. In fact fifteen benefactors in addition to Mr Wishart responded and the fund reached £20,000. The hospital also received in 1881 two-thirds of the revenue from a sum of £16,000. This was given by Miss Airth to fund the Stead Benefaction to open a ward reserved for women and children and to be called the "Stead Medical Ward". A further substantial donation of £8,000 from Miss Elizabeth Waddle in 1888 saw the naming of the Waddle ward. The other medical wards were later named the Struthers ward after Dr James Struthers, a devoted medical officer, president and benefactor of the hospital. In a like manner the Raimes ward, White ward, Watt ward and Hardy wards were named after other benefactors and supporters of the hospital.

Despite the generous gifts, legacies and endowments however the directors were still concerned with the relatively low level of financial support from the general public to produce an adequate ordinary income to meet the everyday running costs of the hospital. In 1872 subscriptions from the public amounted to £408 which amounted to about 2d. per head. Church congregations in particular were singled out for criticism, many being accused of supporting Edinburgh Royal Infirmary and not Leith Hospital.[15]

Staff Changes

To meet the challenge of increasing work and to facilitate advances in medical and nursing practice hospital staffing underwent some important changes in these two decades.

Once again it was Dr Struthers who in January 1874 prodded the directors this time to consider the appointment of a properly qualified Lady Superintendent of Nurses.[16] In November that year Miss E. J. M. McKenzie who had had previous experience in hospital management and the treatment of patients was appointed on a temporary basis. She obviously impressed, as in February 1875 she was formally appointed at a salary of £100 per annum with an apartment and board.[17] This must be considered as the beginning of the high standard of nursing which Leith Hospital has enjoyed in its existence, and also a faltering beginning to nursing training at the hospital.

Nursing training was at that time at an early stage of development. Florence Nightingale after her Crimean experiences inaugurated the Nightingale Training School for Nurses at St Thomas's Hospital, London in 1860 and in Edinburgh an Association for the Training of Nurses was in existence in 1861. Wards in the Royal Infirmary of Edinburgh were set aside for training of probationer nurses in 1862.[18] A tentative approach with regard to nursing training at Leith was made in 1872 when a letter was received from Lady Warrender of Bruntsfield House on behalf of the Institution in Edinburgh for Training Nurses. In it she suggested that one or two of their probationers be trained in Leith Hospital at the expense of the institution.[19] Unfortunately the directors had to reply that they had no accommodation for this purpose but promised to reconsider the matter when additions to buildings were made. With Miss McKenzie's arrival probationers were introduced and conditions agreed for their employment in February 1875.[20] They were to be paid £10 per annum, given board and lodging and a uniform and could be dismissed at any time by the Lady Superintendent for misconduct or negligence. By November of that year however circumstances (certainly financial) changed and probationers were temporarily discontinued and agreement reached that the nursing and auxiliary establishment be as follows.[21]

"Male Ward	Female Wards	Fever Wards
1 day nurse, £30 p.a.	Ditto	Ditto
1 night nurse, £20 p.a.		
1 ward assistant, £14 p.a.		

1 cook, £20 p.a. 1 assistant cook, £12 p.a. 1 housemaid, £18 p.a. 2 porters and Mrs Sutherland and 2 women in the laundry."

Miss Mackenzie was replaced in 1876 as Lady Superintendent by Miss Perry who served until 1892.

Nursing and medical staff were not of course supported at that time by the range of ancillary professions we know now. Patient's diets were the concern of doctors and nurses and "diet tables" were regularly discussed and agreed although none of these survive. The directors were concerned however with the finances particularly when figures were produced indicating that food per occupied bed cost £15 2/8d. in Aberdeen Infirmary, £22 7/3d. in Edinburgh Infirmary and £24 2/6d. in

Leith Hospital! In September 1885 Miss Perry was dispatched to Aberdeen to research the practicalities of feeding patients more cheaply but her report reflected parismony and cheaper butcher meat and milk in Aberdeen rather than profligacy in Leith.[22]

In the 1870s the house surgeon was aided by an assistant and by 1890 an outdoor surgeon had been added to the resident medical staff. By that time also three separate outpatient department medical officers had been added to the seven or eight medical officers. One of these medical officers, Dr Paterson, resigned in 1876. He had served for forty years and was therefore a link with the Dispensary and Casualty Hospital before the opening of Leith Hospital. The beginnings of specialisation were also being seen. The medical officers recognised that medical and surgical work would have to be formally apportioned and in 1880 Dr Garland, Dr Henderson and Dr Hardy agreed to act as physicians and Dr McNair, Dr Finlay and Dr A. R. Coldstream as surgeons. Two years before this in 1878 Dr Struthers had recommended the purchase of a "spray producing machine".[23] This must have been one of Lister's antiseptic sprays which was first recommended publicly by him in 1871. Leith was exercising caution!

In 1884 the volume of dispensing work had increased and the actual dispensing of medicines had become an intolerable burden on the medical officer when the average number of prescriptions per night was forty-five. It was therefore agreed that a part-time dispenser be appointed at a salary of £10 per annum to work between 7 p.m. and 8 p.m. each evening.[24] By 1888 the need for a pathologist was recognised and one appointed but no name appears until 1895 when Dr Theodore Shennon MD is listed.[25]

The consulting surgeons were Professor Spence from 1871-1882 and Patrick Heron Watson who was appointed in 1883 and served until 1908. The consulting physicians during this period were Dr James Struthers from 1884-1891 and Dr John Henderson from 1888-1901.

James Spence (1812-1882) educated at the Royal High School, was appointed surgeon to the Royal Infirmary of Edinburgh in 1854 and to the Chair of Systematic Surgery at Edinburgh in 1864. He was a cautious surgeon and with his constitutional pessimism was known, certainly to his students, as "dismal Jimmy". His *Lectures on Surgery* formed one of the chief textbooks of surgery at that time even though his attitude to Joseph Lister's (his brilliant contemporary) work on antisepsis was to say the least, cautious.[26]

Sir Patrick Heron Watson (1832-1908). An Edinburgh graduate who had been house surgeon to Professor Spence, Heron Watson served as an army surgeon in the Crimean war. He was on the staff of the Royal Infirmary of Edinburgh from 1860 to 1886 and was twice President of the Royal College of Surgeons of Edinburgh. He was one of the most successful surgeons of his time and an excellent teacher with wide interests. He gave whole-hearted support to the movement for the medical education of women and his appointment to Leith Hospital must have given particular pleasure in view of the hospital's role in teaching women medical under-graduates. He was knighted in 1903.[27]

James Struthers (1821-1891) was the eldest of three brothers who qualified in medicine; Alexander the youngest perished at Scutari in the Crimea; John (later Sir John) became Professor of Anatomy at Aberdeen and later President of the Board of Directors of Leith Hospital. James received the gold medal for his MD thesis from Edinburgh University on "The Anatomy and Physiology of the Human Skin". He demonstrated anatomy at the extra-mural school and was assistant pathologist to Edinburgh Royal Infirmary; during the 1847/1848 epidemic of typhus and cholera in Edinburgh he performed 200 post mortem examinations in three months. He became a Fellow of the Royal College of Physicians of Edinburgh in 1861 and was a medical officer to Leith Hospital from 1850-1876. A bachelor he devoted himself to his medical practice but published papers in the Edinburgh Monthly Journal with titles including "On Hydrophobia", "Gangrene of the Lung", and "Acupressure in Amputation of the Thigh". He became consulting physician in 1876 and President of Leith Hospital in 1890 a year before his death, being succeeded by his brother.[28]

John Henderson (1819-1901) born in Jedburgh. Henderson graduated MD at St. Andrews University in 1849 and was elected a Fellow of the Royal College of Surgeons of Edinburgh in 1864. He was in practice in Leith for the whole of his professional life acting as surgeon to Leith Hospital for many years. He took a great interest in local government and entered Leith Town Council in 1871 becoming Provost in 1875 for six years and again in 1885. During this time he was responsible for the Henderson Scheme of Improvement concerned mainly with improved housing and slum clearance. Henderson Street in Leith is his lasting memorial.[29] [30]

Teaching and The Edinburgh School of Medicine for Women

Informal teaching of medical under-graduates at Leith Hospital must have taken place from quite early days. In 1860 one of the house surgeons claimed the fee paid by a student for attending the hospital for six weeks.[31] In 1871 a deputation from the Committee for Securing a Medical Education for Women (the deputation consisting of Professor Masson, Mr Colstone and Dr R. McNair one of the medical officers of Leith Hospital) first requested that the hospital should be made available for the clinical teaching of ladies. The directors seemed sympathetic but felt this might depend on extension of the hospital for which they had no funds at present. The medical officers as a body were however even more discouraging in their opinion that it was "inexpedient to alter the present arrangements of the hospital . . . for the clinical instruction of ladies".[32]

Of course this approach took place before Dr Sophia Jex-Blake, who was to figure prominently in this part of Leith Hospital's, history had graduated Doctor of Medicine at Berne in 1877. She was a vigorous protagonist of the feminist movement and in particular of the struggle to admit women to the practice of medicine. She came to Edinburgh in 1869 and matriculated in the Faculty of Medicine. Although she had many friends and supporters, amongst whom Heron Watson was prominent, she also had implacable enemies who were bitterly opposed to women in medicine and when she was not allowed to complete her studies she brought an action against the University of Edinburgh. Her later qualification abroad and subsequently becoming a Licentiate (1878) and Member (1880) of the Irish College of Physicians allowed her to return to practice in Edinburgh in 1878 and later to set up the Edinburgh Hospital for Women and Children at Bruntsfield Lodge.[33] [34] In 1886 she founded the Edinburgh School of Medicine for Women but problems remained as to which hospital should provide clinical teaching. The Edinburgh Royal Infirmary was unwilling to do so and it was at this point that Leith Hospital entered the scene.

Dr Jex-Blake's approach to Leith Hospital (made initially through Dr Struthers) to provide teaching facilities was, to the hospital's great credit, favourably received. "I should be glad," she wrote, "to make any arrangements as to fees that may be desired by the directors; or if they preferred it would at once guarantee fees to the amount of 200 guineas yearly."[35] Although the lure of financial gain must have attracted the directors it is only fair to say that positive support for Jex-Blake and her ideals was strong both with the directors and the medical officers. In a letter to the secretary of the hospital in May 1886 she set out her requirements which included a daily visit by students to wards and outpatient departments during nine months of the year, two lectures weekly on clinical medicine and surgery in the winter session, appointments as clinical clerks for the students and the admission to operations and post mortem examinations.[36] This was clearly a comprehensive course of clinical instruction. Negotiations proceeded slowly but satisfactorily and the inaugural lecture on "Clinical Instruction" was given by Dr J. Allan Gray on 18th October 1887 [plate 3]. An occasion was made of this, invitations [plate 4] being sent to the Provost of Leith and the baillies, to the Chairmen of the Parochial Boards, medical officers, clergy and to "interested ladies '. The first lecture on clinical surgery and systematic surgery respectively were given by W. A. Finlay FRCSE and C. W. Cathcart, FRCS.

Thus the directors and medical officers of Leith Hospital made possible the first clinical instruction of women students in Edinburgh. Mutual satisfaction was evident; Dr Jex-Blake moved a motion of thanks to the medical officers at the annual meeting of subscribers in 1887[37] and recognition that teaching "added life to the hospital" was made in the director's report of 1892.[38] Unfortunately relationships between all concerned gradually soured although it is difficult to say precisely who was responsible for the deterioration. It is undeniable however that another feminist of strong character and an illustrious female medical graduate Dr Elsie Inglis (commemorated by the Elsie Inglis Hospital in Edinburgh) was involved. Elsie Inglis was one of the first students of the Edinburgh School of Medicine for Women but became involved with others in bitter disagreement and opposition to Jex-Blake. The antagonism may have stemmed from relatively trivial causes.[39] Jex-Blake made it a rule that her students leave Leith Hospital by 5 p.m. but this tended to be disregarded if interesting cases arrived about that time of the day. On 8th June 1888 the women students remained after 5 p.m. to see a patient with a head injury examined. They were asked to leave by Miss Perry, the Lady Superintendent, who received pert replies particularly from Miss Caddell; Jex-Blake's insistence on an apology from her students was disregarded and Miss Caddell and her sister were dismissed from the school for insubordination. The sisters in a "cause celèbre" of the time brought an action for damages of £500 which they won (with reduced damages of £50). Jex-Blake may have been over restrictive in her rules but there is evidence that she was motivated by concern for the well-being of her students in a letter to Dr Gray dated 2nd December 1887. "May I beg you not to keep the class later than 5 p.m." she wrote, "their day begins with a 9 a.m. lecture and they get very tired by evening."[40]

By the following year Dr Jex-Blake was at loggerheads with Dr Gray and the other clinical teachers. Elsie Inglis, as the moving spirit in a group of disaffected women students, was in correspondence with him in an effort to establish another medical school for women. "Many thanks for your letter and for all the trouble you are taking for us," she wrote to Dr Gray on 24th July 1889, "I quite see now that you think a separate school for women a necessity."[41] Eventually the efforts of Elsie Inglis and her father who had influential friends brought about the formation of the Scottish Association for the Medical Education of Women which opened the Medical College for Women as a rival to Jex-Blake's school. The clinical lecturers and the directors of Leith Hospital determined that teaching facilities would be provided for women at Leith irrespective of the school they attended. In 1893 Dr Jex-Blake wrote to the directors setting out conditions on which her school would attend Leith Hospital;[42] they were,

1. That one of the resident medical officers would be a woman selected from among the hospital's old students.
2. That the pathologist at Leith Hospital would be recommended and paid for by the Edinburgh School of Medicine for Women.
3. The Edinburgh School of Medicine for Women would be represented on the Board of Directors.

The directors agreed, with certain provisos, but Dr Jex-Blake was in no mood for any compromise. Considering the early support she had had from Leith Hospital she wrote an extraordinarily antagonistic letter in reply. "If what we ask is not granted," she wrote, "we have fully made up our minds to arrange at once with the Infirmary which offers in several respects very superior attractions to our students and it is not likely that the connection with Leith Hospital once severed will ever be renewed."[43] Professor John Struthers who was at that time President of the Board of Directors felt obliged to write to the directors from his holiday hotel in Harrogate in a somewhat "I told you so" vein. "The letter from Dr Jex-Blake," he wrote, "will open the eyes of the directors to what has all along been evident to me that in the interest of the hospital no such interference can be tolerated."

The Edinburgh School of Medicine for Women closed down in 1898 and the following year Dr Jex-Blake retired to Sussex. The Royal Infirmary of Edinburgh at last opened its doors to women students and women were able to graduate in medicine at Edinburgh University along with men. The story leading up to this civilised ending is darkened by bitterness and recrimination but nothing can diminish the part played by Leith Hospital in enabling women to be taught and to practice medicine.

A Victorian Pot-Pourri

All the major events described occurred against a background of routine hospital work much of which finds a parallel in present times; some matters however have a peculiarly Victorian ambience.

In 1874 Dr McBain, Surgeon to the Royal Navy, requested that since there were no medical facilities for sailors in Royal Navy ships and establishments in the Forth they be admitted to Leith Hospital for treatment. This was agreed at the rate of two shillings per day per sailor, the directors being not averse to increasing revenue.[44] This arrangement continued for many years and there were times when it was used a lot. It was not without its problems as on the occasion in 1884 when "serious misconduct" on the part of several naval patients was reported.[45] It was clear that they had all got outrageously drunk. On the naval authorities being informed action was swift in the form of a telegram from Captain Kennedy, R.N., of H.M.S. "Lord Warden". "Greatly regret conduct of our men," it said, "kindly inform culprits they will be transferred from hospital to jail for six weeks when well enough for removal." The rate of recovery of the men concerned is not recorded!

Patients knew of course that being treated as an inpatient or outpatient they were in receipt of charity. Medical officers were asked to ensure that this charity was appropriate in individual cases. The propriety of free advice and prescriptions was generally related to ability to pay but was sometimes related to the disease being treated. There was some ambivalence about treating venereal disease (except in naval patients)[46] and in 1881 the directors agreed to a suggestion that in cases of venereal disease "wilfully acquired" (!) medicines should be paid for or that a prescription should be given to be obtained by the patients themselves unless unable to pay.[47]

A macabre note was struck by a letter to the medical officers from Dr Andrew Woods, Inspector of Anatomy for Scotland requesting that the bodies of persons dying in the hospital and not claimed by relatives be given over to the anatomical committee in Edinburgh for the purpose of student instruction. This was agreed which was, of course, in line with the law in relation to anatomical dissection at that time.[48]

The directors were also concerned about the length of stay of patients in hospital. Convalescent homes were not directly available to Leith patients at that time although in 1882 a convalescent house for fever patients at Balerno was made available for Leith Hospital patients provided they were "inspected at Edinburgh Fever Hospital".[49] Long stay patients posed problems then as now although from different causes. In October 1887 there were six patients who had been in hospital over three months. One man in hospital sixteen months in whom an operation was impossible was regarded as incurable; it was hoped to have him admitted to Longmore Hospital for Incurables. The other five were not "geriatric"; the diagnoses were urethral fistula and perineal abscesses, favus (a ringworm like infection), tuberculous ascites, contracted joints from acute rheumatism and abdominal aortic aneurysm.[50]

The hospital authorities were also still encumbered by the old Humane Society responsibilities of which the public was well aware. In the 1860s a member of the public had claimed a reward from the directors for saving two boys from drowning in the canal but he was informed there were no funds available for this.[51] But in 1879 the following notice, perhaps regarded as a piece of preventative medicine, was erected at Seafield with similar notices at the Albert Dock, Marine Parade and Annfield, "Bathing from this breakwater is dangerous even to swimmers owing to currents. Leith Hospital August 1879."[52] As late as 1885 the hospital still owned boats, ropes, tackle and life-saving apparatus at Lochend where skating took place during the winter but that year the town council took over the responsibilities and the apparatus.[53]

Nor was this institution free from complaints, justified and otherwise from patients, nor free from squabbles, serious and petty amongst the staff. In 1890 a solicitor's letter claimed £500 damages on behalf of a boy who it was averred had had his big toe amputated unnecessarily and was thereby crippled. Settlement was made on payment of £25![54] In 1879 Dr Campbell complained that Miss Perry, the Lady Superintendent, had discharged patients without his authority — and also denied breakfast to a friend of his![55] Six years later Dr Drever complained of Miss Perry's interference. Incredibly this related to the Lady Superintendent stopping a patient playing the tin whistle except at stated times when he (Dr Drever) desired the patient to "play when he chose".[56] Miss Perry counter-claimed rudeness on the part of Dr Drever! Perhaps more significantly and seriously a letter was sent to the hospital secretary in 1889 by nine nurses claiming they had received "unjust and tyrannical" treatment at the hands of Miss Perry. The first of the signatories resigned and the matter appears to have ended there.

TABLE 1

Cases Treated in Leith Hospital During 1886

SURGICAL CASES	TOTAL
Fracture of skull	5
Fracture of upper jaw and both humeri	1
Fracture of humerus	2
Fracture of humerus (compound)	1
Fracture of radius and ulna	1
Fracture of radius	2
Fracture of phalanges and carpus (compound)	2
Fracture of pelvis (compound)	1
Fracture of femur	12
Fracture of tibia and fibula	4
Fracture of tibia and fibula (compound)	2
Fracture of tibia	4
Fracture of fibula	8
Fracture of ribs	2
Concussion of brain	11
Concussion of spine	2
Diseases of bone	7
Diseases of joints	16
Abscesses	18
Bruises	18
Burns	9
Bursitis	5
Calculus (Vesical)	1
Carbuncle	2
Cellulitis	2
Cut throat	2
Ear	2
Eye	2
Haemorrhoids	2
Hernia (Strangulated, Femoral)	1
Hydrocele	1
Phymosis	2
Sprains	6
Stricture	4
Ulcers	3
Varicose veins	1

Venereal	14
Wounds	23
	201

MEDICAL CASES

Alimentary system	21
Circulator system	19
Respiratory system	77
Nervous system	18
Haemopoietic system	4
Genito-Urinary system	15
Integumentary system	3
Alcoholism	22
Rheumatism	22
Carcinoma	6
Scorbutus	4
Croup	2
Ague	1
Submersions	11
Opium poisoning	6
Irritant poisoning	1
	232

FEVER CASES

Typhoid	29
Typhus	21
Scarlatina	25
Measles	14
Smallpox	26
Febricula	9
Erysipelas	7
Diphtheria	1
Ague	3
Cerebro-Spinal Fever	1
Various	18
	154

TOTAL SURGICAL DEATHS	14
TOTAL MEDICAL DEATHS	22
TOTAL FEVER DEATHS	16

REFERENCES

CHAPTER 3

1. Leith Hospital Annual Report. 1871.
2. Ibid., 1890.
3. Leith Hospital Board of Directors Minutes 5.10.1871.
4. Leith Hospital Annual Report. 1890.
5. Ibid., 1877.

6.   Ibid., 1890.
7.   Leith Hospital Board of Directors, Minutes 7.1.1873.
8.   Marshall, J. S. Op. cit. p. 11.
9.   Memorandum to Provost, Magistrates and Town Council of Leith 16.12.1881.
10.   Letter to Leith Town Council 6.11.1888.
11.   Leith Hospital Board of Directors, Minutes 6.12.1888.
12.   Ibid., 24.10.1870.
13.   Ibid., 30.3.1875.
14.   Ibid., 4.4.1875.
15.   Marshall, J. S. Op. cit. p. 12.
16.   Leith Hospital Board of Directors, Minutes 12.1.1874.
17.   Ibid., 4.2.1875.
18.   Logan-Turner, A. (1937). *The Story of a Great Hospital; Royal Infirmary of Edinburgh.* p. 210. Edinburgh: Oliver & Boyd.
19.   Leith Hospital Board of Directors, Minutes 31.7.1872.
20.   Ibid., 13.2.1875.
21.   Ibid., 10.11.1875.
22.   Ibid., 30.12.1880.
23.   Ibid., 9.8.1878.
24.   Ibid., 12.6.1884.
25.   Leith Hospital Annual Report, 1895.
26.   Comrie, J. D. Op. cit. p. 673.
27.   Ross, J. A. (1978). *The Edinburgh School of Surgery after Lister.* p. 11. Edinburgh: Churchill-Livingstone.
28.   *Edinburgh Medical Journal* (1891). Vol. 37. p. 90.
29.   *Leith Observer* 6.7.1901.
30.   *Medical Directory*, 1881.
31.   Leith Hospital Board of Directors, Minutes 3.7.1860.
32.   Ibid., 6.4.1871.
33.   Comrie, J. D. Op. cit. pp. 667-669.
34.   *Who Was Who* (1920). Vol. 1. p. 380.
35.   Todd, M. *The Life of Sophia Jex-Blake* (1918). p. 497. London: MacMillan & Co.
36.   Leith Hospital Board of Directors, Minutes 13.5.1886.
37.   Leith Hospital Annual Report, 1887. p. 380.
38.   Leith Hospital Annual Report, 1892.
39.   Lawrence, M. *Shadow of Swords* (1971). p. 53. London: Michael Joseph.
40.   Personal Papers, Dr J. D. A. Gray.
41.   Ibid.
42.   Leith Hospital Board of Directors, Minutes 15.9.1893.
43.   Ibid., 21.9.1893.
44.   Ibid., 6.4.1874.
45.   Ibid., 9.2.1884.
46.   Ibid., 1.12.1877.
47.   Ibid., 9.6.1881.
48.   Ibid., 4.2.1875.
49.   Ibid., 14.7.1882.
50.   Ibid., 22.9.1887.
51.   Ibid., 21.1.1861.

52.   Ibid., 14.8.1879.
53.   Ibid., 8.10.1885.
54.   Ibid., 9.10.1890.
55.   Ibid., 9.2.1879.
56.   Ibid., 13.11.1885.
57.   Ibid., 5.12.1889.

Expansion and Specilisation. 1891-1910

Someone in the 1870s hoping to see substantial improvement in social conditions in two decades time must have been grievously disappointed. Conditions in Leith in the years between 1894 and 1901 have been graphically described by a doctor who knew them at first hand. Doctor (later Sir) Leslie MacKenzie succeeded Dr J. Allan Gray as the first full time Medical Officer of Health for Leith in 1894. Speaking in 1928 he described the Port of Leith as one of the great gateways of infection from all other countries of the world, infection which found its way into the old lanes full of people "many on the margin of poverty and some far below it". "I have seen," he said, "in a miserable garret with hardly a bed where a father was almost dying of hunger with his son lying dead on a miserable mattress and when I looked at the son I found that almost half his face had been eaten off by rats." His notebooks were full, he was reported as saying, of cases of destitution, disease of every variety and meetings with people from the common lodging houses and dens.[1] It was with such a social background therefore that Leith Hospital saw the end of the 19th century and the beginning of the 20th.

Continuing Problems with Zymotic Diseases

Mention has already been made of Dr J. Allan Gray's criticism of the hospital and the Town Council's eventual success in establishing a fever hospital. Dr Gray was in a somewhat difficult position. He was a medical officer of the hospital from 1881 to 1891 and was Leith's first Medical Officer of Health on a part-time basis from 1886 until his resignation in 1894. It was clear that he, very properly, looked on his role as the person responsible for the control of infection in the burgh as a vital one but his vigorous efforts to achieve this goal were not always appreciated by the hospital authorities. At the annual meeting of the Friends and Subscribers of Leith Hospital in 1890 Dr Gray had asked leave to make a statement which was to the effect that accommodation at the disposal of the hospital for the treatment and isolation of infectious diseases was quite inadequate and he also made charges of maladministration.[2] He followed this up with a report extending to forty manuscript pages to the Town Council which did not mince matters and which created something of a sensation. It criticised the directors for apportioning the oldest and most unsatisfactory part of the hospital for fever patients, for mismanagement and for being responsible for the overworking of nurses. Comments in and letters to the local

36

press were uninhibited and were equally so in the national medical and nursing journals. The *Medical Press* of the 13th May 1891 said, "If the facts are as above indicated, and there is no need to doubt their substantial accuracy, nothing short of a government enquiry is indicated"; and later, "The Medical Officer's report reads like a page from the chronicle of some medieval writer not like a picture of any possible occurrence in the year of our Lord 1891".[3] From a vantage point of distance in time the directors may be seen as not exclusively responsible for the situation, saddled as they were by financial constraints and unaided by a Town Council which was tardy in meeting its full responsibilities. The Secretary of the hospital prepared for the directors a memorandum to enable them to consider the charges made by Dr Gray. It pointed out the scarcity of nurses in Edinburgh and Leith for the previous eighteen months and gives the impression of a devoted staff coping to the best of their abilities with a rush of typhus and scarlatina patients in less than ideal premises.[4] The directors continued of course to press the Town Council for action, the lack of which they deplored in a letter in September 1892 which gave a definite ultimatum — "having regard to the limited accommodation at their disposal and the impossibility of proper isolation they will *not* receive the town's fever patients into their hospital after 1st October 1893."[5] The Council had indeed purchased in 1891 old school premises in South Fort Street and converted them for use as an infectious diseases hospital but this was another makeshift and inadequate building. In 1893-1894 the community of Leith had another severe epidemic to cope with, this time of smallpox and the Council had a temporary wooden hospital built on Leith Links. From November 1893 to August 1894, 384 patients from Leith were admitted to hospital with this disease of whom fifty died including seven children.[6] Therefore before the felicitous opening of the Burgh Fever Hospital at East Pilton the Council was in the absurd position of having premises for infectious diseases at King Street, South Fort Street, Leith Links and 18 Coal Hill (which had been purchased in 1885 to accommodate cholera victims in an emergency).[7]

Further Extensions to the Hospital

In the 1890s there was more than one argument for extending the hospital and increasing the number of beds. In 1893 Dr Elder one of the physicians to the hospital produced a pamphlet arguing that on the basis of population, what was available in similar towns elsewhere in Scotland and the increase in volume and diversity of medical work undertaken, Leith Hospital should have a complement of 153 beds instead of the 59 at that time.[8] In 1893 the last year that fever patients were admitted as such, 992 inpatients were treated and 7,983 outpatients attended. Three years later a similar number of inpatients were treated (999) but they included 85 gynaecology and 30 eye patients and outpatient attendances had risen to 11,774.[9] Another reason for increasing the number of beds related to the teaching of medical undergraduate students. It will be remembered that 1893 was the year that saw Dr Jex Blake and her medical school for women in conflict with the directors and medical officers of Leith Hospital. It was the same year that the directors received an intimation from the Medical Board of the Scottish Triple Qualification (LRCPE, LRCSE, LRFPSG), that recognition of the hospital would cease unless the number of beds available for general cases was raised to 80.[10] The directors were doubtful whether additions to the hospital were justified on this basis and they thought that an increase in expenditure was unlikely to be met by student fees. They had meetings with the managers of Edinburgh Royal Infirmary to try to agree on the sharing of teaching of women students but the Board of the Triple Qualification would not recognise combined instruction at the two hospitals.[11] Despite the difficulties however and with the enthusiastic support of medical staff the directors saw the advantages in having a hospital recognised for teaching purposes. Their first step was the conversion of the old "Fever House" for general cases but allowing for rearranging and enlarging the dispensary department and providing additional accommodation for nurses and servants.[12] By 1894 the original 1848-1851 hospital building which had been raised to three storeys was being called the "West House" and the 1873-1875 extension, the "East House". The disposition of beds was as follows:

	Medical: Male	Medical: Female	Total
West House	12 (1 ward)	12 (1 ward)	
East House	14 (2 wards)		38
	Surgical: Male	Surgical: Female	
East House	28 (4 wards)	14 (2 wards)	42
			80
West House	"Observation"		3
East House	"Observation"/Staff		3
			86

The necessity for further extension in the 1890s was recognised by the formation of a "committee as to the increase in beds" in 1896. Some members were of the opinion that bed numbers could be increased by "planning in each ward its full complement of beds";[13] in other words by cramming more beds in. It was eventually agreed however that a scheme for 100 beds should be pursued[14] and it was perhaps fortunate that Queen Victoria's Diamond Jubilee celebrations were very much in the minds of citizens at that time. The Town Council initially suggested that this event should be marked by the provision of a convalescent home for the people of Leith but at a meeting of representative townspeople it was proposed that a public appeal be launched for £12,000 (to which sum the hospital would contribute £2,000) to extend the hospital to a bed complement of 100.[15] The appeal and the

ON

CLINICAL INSTRUCTION.

A LECTURE

INTRODUCTORY TO THE FIRST COURSE OF

CLINICAL MEDICINE

IN CONNECTION WITH

THE EDINBURGH SCHOOL OF MEDICINE FOR WOMEN.

DELIVERED AT LEITH HOSPITAL,
ON 18TH OCTOBER 1887.

BY

J. ALLAN GRAY, M.A., M.D., F.R.C.P.ED.

LEITH: GARDNER BROTHERS.

1887.

PLATE 3. Frontispiece of the first lecture given at Leith Hospital in 1887 by Dr J. A. Gray in connection with the Edinburgh School of Medicine for Women

Edinburgh School of Medicine for Women,

IN ASSOCIATION WITH

THE LEITH HOSPITAL.

The EXECUTIVE COMMITTEE invite the presence of

AT THE

OPENING LECTURE

ON CLINICAL MEDICINE,

TO BE DELIVERED BY

DR ALLAN GRAY, F.R.C.P.,

At 4 p.m. on Tuesday, October 18th, 1887,

AT THE LEITH HOSPITAL.

SOPHIA JEX-BLAKE, M.D.,
Hon. Sec. of the School.

PLATE 4. Invitation card to the opening lecture from Dr Sophia Jex-Blake

surrounding publicity helped to focus attention on the hospital at an important time. This attention was perhaps required in the light of a wry comment in the annual report of 1896. "In these days when Nansen is discovering the North Pole it is a lamentable fact that some persons exist in Leith who have not yet discovered Leith Hospital". The services of an architect, Mr W. N. Thomson were engaged in 1898. He prepared plans for a large Renaissance block of three storeys to the south of existing buildings, facing King Street and on a site previously purchased by the hospital. These new buildings were fitted with electric light, an innovation soon extended to the rest of the hospital. At the same time and on the opposite (i.e. east) side of King Street a new nurses home, kitchen and laundry were built and connected to the main hospital by a subway. The total cost of these major extensions was approximately £24,000 but this was adequately covered by donations. The new buildings [plate 5] were formally opened on 22nd May 1903 by the Earl of Leven and Melville the Lord High Commissioner of that year's General Assembly of the Church of Scotland.[16] On the exterior east facing wall of the new pavilion is a medallion of Queen Victoria with the inscription — "This pavilion was erected in commemoration of the Diamond Jubilee of Her Majesty Queen Victoria, May 1897."

With the completion of the new block some reconstruction of the "East House" was carried out so that the disposition of beds was now as follows:[17]

King Street Pavilion

1st Floor (Ground)	Large ward. Male surgical.	18
	Small ward. Nurses sick room.	4
2nd Floor	*Large ward. [Female Surgical	16
	[Female Ophthalmic	2
	Small ward. Gynaecological	6
3rd Floor	Large ward. [Male surgical	16
	[Male ophthalmic	2
Corner Block		
	Large ward. Female medical.	16
West House		
	Two wards. Male medical.	23
	Observation ward.	2

*[plate 6]   105

This, with the exception of the post 1914/18 war children's wing extension was the form in which the hospital largely functioned for most of its remaining existence as an acute inpatient hospital.

There was another addition to the hospital's facilities which deserves mention. In 1901 Mrs Jessie Currie purchased and fitted up a

Cottage Home in Corstorphine, provided a qualified matron and intimated she would pay all expenses of maintenance for a period. This was for the reception of suitable persons requiring rest during convalescence. Suitable persons it was stipulated, however, did not include those with infections, consumption, skin diseases, epilepsy, mental disease or children requiring assistance with dressing. "I place at your disposal," she wrote to the directors, "six beds" and the offer was cordially accepted.[18] A greatly appreciated amenity, this convalescent home was available to patients from Leith Hospital for many years.

An improvement in the hospital's amenity was made in 1908 when the site that had been occupied by South Leith Poorhouse was purchased by the hospital. The poorhouse was moved to Seafield and the vacant site became the Taylor Gardens.[19]

Finances and Change of Constitution

The building extensions were made possible by good responses to special appeals for funds but the directors still had the predicament of meeting increasing everyday running costs. In 1896 and 1906 ordinary income and ordinary expenditure was respectively £2716 and £4078 and £3347 and £5995[20] showing an increasing annual deficit which had to be met on occasions by realising securities. In 1906 ordinary income derived from donations, subscriptions and collections and included donations of £100 from the Leith Dock Commission, £150 from Leith Parish Council and £50 from the Town Council; in the same year investments amounted to £22,950. At that time the cost per patient per day was 2/9d. and the cost per bed was £50 7/9d. which was less than that of the Edinburgh Royal Infirmary.

There had been an increase in the number of patients treated but not a parallel rise in donations. In the 1890s the local churches again came in for particular criticism, the President of the Board of Directors deprecating the continuing practice in some congregations in Leith of taking collections for Edinburgh Royal Infirmary. A charity, he thought, should begin at home.[21] Also, in 1894 there was no income from the medical school.[22] All items of expenditure were carefully scrutinised; it was recommended that the practice of other dispensaries be instituted at Leith and one penny be charged for a prescription; vaccination by hospital staff was stopped except for children whose parents were unable to pay.[23] In 1908 the medical officers in commenting on the large increase in outpatient attendances, were of the opinion that this was largely due to the depressed condition of trade; at the same time they thought a certain number of patients did not require treatment at a *charitable* institution.[24] Two years later they reported a considerable decrease in medical and gynaecological outpatients which they ascribed to the action of the hospital in issuing schedules enquiring into the circumstances of those seeking advice.[25] In other words some kind of means test was being applied. A happier note was struck in 1904 when the directors were able to thank the Town Council for embodying in a recent act of parliament a clause relieving hospitals from payment of Burgh assessment. Again, a happy though poignant event in 1907 was the donation of £500 to the hospital by Herr Knoblauch the German consul in Leith which the chairman at the annual meeting of the General Court of Contributors called "cementing the union between the two nations".

The directors by 1905 were recognising the disadvantages of not having an up-to-date constitution (the original had been framed in 1850) and a set of rules for the better management of the hospital and employment of staff. They were also anxious to give direct representation on the Board to several public bodies of importance in the town. The constitutions of several similar institutions in Scotland were considered. The Western Infirmary of Glasgow which had been incorporated under the Company's Act was approached about the cost and advantages of incorporation and the answers provided persuaded the directors to pursue this end.[27] The matter came to a successful conclusion in 1907 when the hospital became "Leith Hospital (incorporated)" with a President and Vice President, sixteen "Managers" instead of Directors and an Honorary Secretary and Honorary Treasurer. This was the managerial structure which functioned until the advent of the National Health Service in 1948.

The Staffing of the Hospital

At the time of opening of the King Street Pavilion the staff of the hospital with the exception of the visiting and honorary medical staff was as follows:

Resident medical staff — 5
Matron — 1
Night Superintendent — 1
Nurses — 33
Maids, laundry and kitchen staff — 15
Porters — 3
Engineer — 1
Fireman — 1
Sewing maid — 1[28]

As has been indicated visiting medical staff, allocated medical and surgical work to themselves in 1880. In 1883 assistant medical officers had been appointed to work in the outpatient department and in 1888 they were appointed specifically as outpatient department medical officers. The march of specialisation continued in 1897 when physicians and surgeons were appointed with these titles. Assistant physicians and surgeons were appointed in 1902 to cope with the outpatient work but they were soon requesting access to beds quoting the practice in other places particularly London teaching hospitals and six beds each were allocated to the senior assistant physician and surgeon.[29] The appointment of assistants to the posts of physicians or surgeons became customary and it was also quite common for physicians and surgeons, assistants or otherwise to be appointed to senior posts in the Edinburgh Royal Infirmary. In many respects therefore Leith Hospital was regarded as a stepping stone to posts in the Infirmary and for this reason some very eminent names appear in the lists of Leith Hospital medical staff. Consulting physicians and surgeons continued to be appointed from the ranks of retiring physicians and surgeons of the hospital but the posts were also used as a way of honouring other eminent medical men.

Consulting physicians during the period in question were G. W. Balfour, Claude Muirhead and Alexander Bruce. The Consulting surgeon was William Stewart.

George William Balfour (1823-1903) was a lecturer in Medicine at the University from 1866 and became eminent as a specialist in diseases of the heart. His *"Clinical Lectures on Diseases of the Heart and Aorta"* and *"The Senile Heart"* were classical monographs of their time. He was President of the Royal College of Physicians of Edinburgh from 1882-1884 and the first physician to the Royal Edinburgh Hospital for Incurables (now Longmore Hospital). The honour of Physician in ordinary to His Majesty Edward VII was accorded to him. He was an uncle of the writer Robert Louis Stevenson. He had had some contact with Leith Hospital as chairman of the Edinburgh School of Medicine for Women in 1889.[30] [31]

Claude Muirhead (1836-1910) was physician to the Edinburgh Royal Infirmary, consultant physician to the Edinburgh Fever Hospital and also to Chalmers Hospital. He became one of the first authorities on life insurance. A much respected Fellow of the Royal College of Physicians of Edinburgh, he twice refused the Presidency of that College.[32] [33]

Alexander Bruce (1854-1911). He became a lecturer in pathology at Surgeons Hall and pathologist at the Edinburgh Royal Infirmary. His special interest was neurology one of his main works being the *"Topographical Atlas of the Spinal Cord"*. He later became physician and clinical lecturer in the Royal Infirmary. As well as being a Fellow of the Royal College of Physicians of Edinburgh he was elected to the Fellowship of the Royal Society of Edinburgh and was given the honorary degree of Doctor of Laws of St. Andrews University.[34] [35]

William Stewart (?1852-?). He graduated MB in Edinburgh in 1875 and obtained the gold medal for his MD thesis in 1879. He became a Fellow of the Royal College of Surgeons of Edinburgh in 1897 but rather unusually took a BSc in public health in 1876 and the Fellowship of the Royal Faculty of Physicians and Surgeons, Glasgow in 1882. He had studied in Vienna before becoming physician for diseases of the eye at Anderson's College Dispensary, Glasgow and then surgeon at Leith Hospital.[36] [37]

Appointed as physicians during this time were William Elder and H. G. Langwill.

William Elder (1865-1931). After qualifying in Edinburgh in 1885 he was house physician at Edinburgh Royal Infirmary and later came to Leith as assistant and then partner to Dr James Struthers. He was a medical officer at Leith Hospital for fifteen years first to the outpatient department and then inpatients and finally as physician. He was awarded the gold medal for his MD thesis *"Aphasia and the Cerebral Speech Mechanism"* which was published as a book in 1897. He became a recognised authority in neurology and examined in this subject for the membership of the Royal College of Physicians of Edinburgh to which he was elected a Fellow in 1894. Deafness caused him some incapacity in later years but he continued to write, publishing *"The Physical Basis of Memory"* in 1900 and *"Studies in Psychology"* in 1927.[38] He clearly enjoyed travel and in 1898 donated £50 to Leith Hospital funds proceeds from his public lecture on a recent visit to Russia.[39]

Hamilton Graham Langwill (1868-1946). Dr Langwill was in general practice for forty-five years. Graduating MB at Edinburgh in 1889 and MD in 1898 he became a Fellow of the Royal College of Physicians of Edinburgh in 1896. He served as medical officer and physician to Leith Hospital from 1897 to 1912 and during the 1914-18 war served as a captain RAMC with the 2nd Scottish General Hospital. He lectured at the Leith Nautical College for many years. A cultivated man, interested in music and literature, he was something of an authority on churches and cathedrals which he visited and photographed frequently.[40]

One of the assistant medical officers appointed from 1903 to 1909 was Edwin Bramwell, eldest son of Sir Byrom Bramwell and a future Professor of clinical medicine at Edinburgh and President of the Royal College of Physicians of Edinburgh.

Around the turn of the century three surgeons were appointed, William Stewart in 1897, already referred to as a consulting surgeon, Alexander Miles in the same year and A. A. Scot-Skirving in 1904.

Alexander Miles (1865-1953). Qualifying in 1888 he was elected a Fellow of the Royal College of Surgeons of Edinburgh in 1890. Following his appointment as surgeon at Leith Hospital he became assistant surgeon and surgeon at the Edinburgh Royal Infirmary until his retirement. He wrote with Professor Alexis Thomson the renowned *"Manual of Surgery"* and also a textbook of *"Operative Surgery"*. He became President of the Royal College of Surgeons of Edinburgh. The University of Edinburgh conferred on him the degree of Doctor of Laws following his work as a member of the University Court.[41]

Archibald Adam Scot-Skirving CMG. (1869-1930). As was common practice he resigned his post as surgeon to Leith Hospital to become surgeon at Edinburgh Royal Infirmary. His first association with Leith Hospital however had been as a house surgeon in 1894 and he was later medical officer to the outpatient department. He was one of those who served in the 1914/18 war as well as in the South African war when he was chief surgeon to the Imperial Yeomanry Field Hospital and was awarded the CMG. for his work in relation to this. He had some unorthodox habits. It is recorded that he sucked formalin tablets when operating and rode a scooter between his wards in the Royal Infirmary.[42] [43]

Further moves towards providing specialist services at the hospital were made in 1896 when an ophthalmic surgeon and gynaecologist were appointed following representations by the Medical Staff Committee in 1895.[44] The community had recognised the need for these services as a Leith Eye Dispensary had been established at 102 Kirkgate in 1891. The following year a combined Dispensary for Diseases of the Eye and Diseases of Women was opened at 56 Bridge Street.[45] The ophthalmic surgeon associated with the Dispensary **William George Sym** (1864-1938) who lectured in the Extramural School of Medicine became the first ophthalmic surgeon to Leith Hospital. Later he became ophthalmic surgeon to the Royal Infirmary of Edinburgh, consulting surgeon to Scottish Command of the army and was author of a well-known book on *"Diseases and Injuries of the Eye"*. He was appointed consulting ophthalmic surgeon to Leith Hospital in 1906.[46] He was succeeded by **Arthur H. H. Sinclair** (1867-1962) who introduced the technique of quantitative perimetry and introduced to Edinburgh in 1922 the operation of intracapsular extraction of the lens. He became consulting ophthalmic surgeon at Leith Hospital in 1912.[47]

The first physician for diseases peculiar to women was D. Berry Hart. He was succeeded in 1900 by N. T. Brewis and by J. H. Ferguson.

David Berry Hart (1851-1920). Graduated at Edinburgh in 1877 and only three years later published his work *"A Structural Anatomy of the Female Pelvic Floor"*, and with Dr Freeland Barber he wrote a very widely known *"Manual of Gynaecology"*. He left Leith Hospital to become gynaecologist at the Edinburgh Royal Infirmary. His portrait hangs in the hall of the Royal College of Physicians of Edinburgh of which he was a Fellow and also Honorary Librarian from 1902-1920.[48] [49]

Nathaniel Thomas Brewis (1856-1924). After his association with Leith Hospital he became gynaecologist at Edinburgh Royal Infirmary. His textbook *"Outlines of Gynaecological Diagnoses"* was well regarded in its time. A Fellow of both the Royal Colleges of Physicians and Surgeons of Edinburgh he was a noted sportsman and was a Scottish rugby internationalist.[50]

James Haig Ferguson (1863-1934). A Fellow of the Royal College of Physicians of Edinburgh and the Royal College of Surgeons of Edinburgh his name was for long associated with the care of the unmarried mother and her child. He had been a family doctor for twenty years and only after obtaining his first hospital appointment as gynaecologist to Leith Hospital did he graduate by steps to specialist practice. With W. F. N. Haultain he wrote *"A Handbook of Obstetric Nursing"* and contributed to the *"Combined Textbook of Obstetrics and Gynaecology"*. He was credited with getting the first antenatal outpatient clinic started in Britain. A member of the Royal Company of Archers (the Sovereign's bodyguard in Scotland), he was elected President of the Royal College of Surgeons of Edinburgh in 1929.[51]

Röntgen directed attention to the diagnostic value of x-rays in 1896 and in the same year Edinburgh Royal Infirmary established an electrical department. There is a record of a fee of one guinea being paid to Dr Dawson Turner, medical electrician to the Royal Infirmary and one of the first to recognise the importance of x-rays, for a Röntgen ray photograph of a patient in Leith Hospital in 1901.[52] Later that year Dr Turner's advice was sought on what apparatus should be installed in Leith Hospital and in 1903 Frederick Gardiner was appointed the first "medical electrician". X-ray, high frequency and Faradic apparatus was obtained at a cost of £257. Dr Gardiner was followed in 1906 by F. R. Kerr and in that year this department had taken fifty-six "photographs" and had conducted 168 x-ray examinations. It was also as has been implied responsible for the application of various forms of electricity including high frequency and "switchboard".

Mention has already been made of the appointment of a pathologist in 1897. The first incumbent was Theodore Shennan who left in 1903 and later became Professor of Pathology at Aberdeen. Pathologists came and went quite rapidly and up to 1910 Shennan was followed by W. T. Ritchie (who later became Professor of Medicine at Edinburgh and President of the Royal College of Physicians of Edinburgh), J. D. Comrie (future author of *"A History of Scottish Medicine"*) and Lindsay S. Milne.

A further medical post was established in 1901, that of medical registrar, the first incumbent being Dr John Easson. This post had clinical duties but also required the incumbent to keep records and produce statistics.

Unfortunately the appointment of junior hospital staff was a matter which caused some bitterness between directors and senior medical staff about this time. The first female house officer, Dr Marion Ritchie died of typhus in 1890 as has been recorded and the second, Dr Alice MacLaren (MB London), was appointed in 1891. These events would seem entirely compatible with the director's and medical officer's support for the medical education of women. Nevertheless the doctors were unhappy with the second appointment. Although they pointed out in a letter to the directors that they "almost unanimously" favoured admission of ladies to the profession, a view founded on the "undeniable principle that women ought to have the right of choosing medical advisers of their own sex," they went on to say that they resented the violation of the principle "as is involved in the appointment of a woman as a house physician to a mixed hospital". The logic of this is difficult to follow but the real objection may be revealed in a later sentence to the effect that they "cannot but protest against our latest unanimous recommendations for the post of house physician being departed from by the directors".[53] However the surgeons of the hospital wrote to the directors a letter which contained a surprising statement, "Such cases [serious accidents, urgent surgical emergencies and submersion cases] fall to be treated by the lady resident who is necessarily unfit to attend to many of them effectively." They requested the appointment of a fourth resident. The directors refused to alter their decision pointing out that Dr MacLaren's qualifications were surgical as well as medical. Skill and competence of women medical graduates soon became undeniable even to the most bigoted of critics and their devotion was surely never in doubt. Another young house officer Dr Mabel Ross was to die during the tenure of her post of typhoid fever in 1904.*

Friction between the two parties continued and culminated in 1896 in the resignation of five of the medical officers. The press reported these troubles fairly extensively. One of the reasons for this most unhappy state of affairs was the continuing mode of appointment of house officers; in Edinburgh Royal Infirmary the visiting staff selected the candidates, the managers merely exercising the formality of appointment whereas in Leith Hospital the directors claimed the right of selection.[54] Another matter which precipitated at least one of the resignations was the performance in the hospital of a gynaecological operation by a doctor not on the staff of Leith Hospital.[55] The medical officer who had requested this intervention defended himself by claiming that the patient concerned would not go to the Infirmnary and that he had not sufficient experience of the particular operation to perform it.[56] The directors considered he should have approached the consulting surgeon of the hospital but as the medical officer pointed out he (the consulting surgeon) was not a gynaecologist.

As is not infrequent the eventual outcome of these disagreements was beneficial, a system of junior appointments similar to the Edinburgh Royal Infirmary being adopted and a gynaecologist to the hospital appointed.

The nursing staff was now far removed from the questionable image of the early days of the hospital. Photographs of the Lady Superintendent and groups of nurses taken around 1896 show neatly uniformed, intelligent young women who by that time were receiving a comprehensive and structured training [plates 7 & 8]. In the early 1900s as has already been mentioned the nursing staff consisted of thirty-

---

*Dr Ross's father presented a microscope to the hospital which is still in the possession of the Lothian Health Board. It has the following inscription. "This microscope was given for the use of the resident physicians in Leith Hospital by Mr A. Ellison Ross as a remembrance of his daughter Mabel Ross MB, ChB who while assistant house physician died in the hospital on 11th September 1904."

three nurses not including the Lady Superintendent and Night Superintendent. A decade before only thirteen were employed[57] and conditions when the "Fever House" was part of the hospital were far from
satisfactory. Nurses had to sleep and eat in the same room which was
recognised as being detrimental to their well being especially in times
of epidemic.[58] Training was sufficiently organised in the hospital for the
Lady Superintendent to accept for training for two years a probationer
from the Scottish Branch of the Queen Victoria Jubilee Institute for
Nurses. Medical officers were providing lectures to nurses in 1894 and
money was being allocated ro provide prizes for nurses examined on
the lectures given by the medical officers.[59] £8 was spent on a skeleton
for the instruction of nurses in 1899.[60] In the previous year the training
period had been raised to three from two years although those already
trained in a fever or children's hospital needed to complete only two
years. The salaries for probationers then were, first year £10, second
year £15 and third year £18 per annum plus of course board and uni-
forms.[61] In 1907 an approach from the Royal British Nurses Association in London[62] indicating the intention to grant diplomas on completing three years training and passing an examination met with coopera-
tion by the managers and by that year Leith Hospital nurses were so
well regarded that they were sought as private nurses. The Matron was
empowered to supply nurses if available and the cases appeared suitable and stringent rules of conduct were laid down. The charge varied
from £1.10/- to two guineas per week but two and a half guineas were
charged for infectious cases.[63] Nurses were also expected to undertake
procedures now under the aegis of other health professionals. At the
beginning of the century money was allotted to provide tuition for
nurses in the massage treatment of surgical cases.[64]

The Changing Pattern of Work

The general increase in most aspects of the hospital's work can be
seen from table 2 and some idea of the type of cases dealt with on an
inpatient basis from table 3. No record exists of the type of surgical
operations carried out at this time.

The problem of infectious diseases obviously became much less
important for the hospital after the opening of the Burgh Fever Hospital in 1896. Concern persisted however with the continuing and important problem of tuberculosis. The danger of infection from cases of
open pulmonary tuberculosis both for other patients and members of
staff were well recognised and it was resolved on the basis of a report by
the physicians in 1904 that cases of "phthisis pulmonalis" would no
longer be admitted except when they required treatment for some
other condition.[65] Other clinical problems causing disquiet amongst
the staff were those associated with alcohol abuse — problems not
unknown in modern times. In 1892 it was requested that alcoholic
cases should not be admitted unless on Dr Garland's (one of the medi-

cal officers) special request.[66] Three years later the medical officers recommended that all ordinary cases of alcohol poisoning ought to be treated but that "no accommodation should be offered for cases of delirium tremens or insanity which would require the keeping of a male and female attendant".[67] An account of the dispensary department written by one of the residents in 1896 includes the following. "The whole staff, doctors, nurses and porters, occasionally have their patience and good-will severely tried by cases of alcoholism whose grossly insulting language and violent behaviour rendered them most undesirable patients. Where it is necessary to retain such in hospital for treatment the head of the police force will on application permit the attendance of a constable so long as the patient is violent or abusive. Such cases are no longer permitted into the ordinary wards but are placed in the isolation wards where their noisy behaviour does not annoy the other patients."

In the same publication comment is made with regard to some aspects of patient care which has a flavour of the time. The accepted proximity of cleanliness to godliness is seen in the sentence "Anyone watching certain cases as they are carried into the outpatients department cannot but be struck on seeing the same persons a few hours afterwards in the wards by the marked change in their appearance produced by a judicious use of water and finished off by clean bedclothes and a brush and comb." And as regards patients' views on hospital food — "One will consider he is overfed while another complains of starvation; the truth being that under strict medical orders both are receiving as much food as is good for their particular ailment. In the majority of cases the food supplied both as to quality and cooking forms a more suitable diet than the same individuals could have received at their own homes."[68]

The dispensary and outpatient work was by that time organised on the basis of the following intimation to the public:

"Medical cases	Every week day at 9.30 a.m.
Surgical cases	Monday, Tuesday, Thursday and Friday at 9.30 a.m.
Eye cases	Tuesday and Friday at 5 p.m.
Women	Monday and Thursday at 4 p.m.
Dressings	Every weekday at 9.30 a.m.
Teeth extracted	Every day at 7 p.m.
Accident and Emergencies	All hours of day and night.

Names of those unable to come to the Dispensary must be given by 8.45 a.m.

Only urgent cases on Sundays.

Medicines dispensed every week day 10 a.m.-12 and 6-7 p.m."

It was in this year, 1906, that gratuitous vaccination ceased at the hospital since it was provided by public authorities.

A Miscellany of Events

There was no doubt that by the beginning of this century the community of Leith had a hospital of which it could be justly proud. Nurses received a training which could equal that obtained in much larger hospitals and the visiting medical and surgical staff were men of eminence for the reasons already mentioned. In his letter of resignation Dr Elder wrote in 1909 thanking the directors for "opportunities of scientifically studying disease in its many forms which only a thoroughly modern and up-to-date hospital such as Leith now possesses, is capable of affording".[69] The junior staff was also generally of high quality. The Registrar in 1910, Dr T. Addis, left Leith Hospital to take up the post of assistant Professor of Medicine at Stanford University, San Francisco.[70] One of the visiting staff wrote in 1896 "The position of the resident doctor is also a coveted one amongst junior members of the profession. Only in such posts can young medical men acquire that wide experience in management, in diagnosis and in the treatment of disease which is so necessary to a successful doctor. From the varied nature of cases met with and the vicinity to the Edinburgh School, Leith Hospital is able to choose for its residents some of the more skilful and cultivated young graduates." And later he made a general comment on hospital treatment which he clearly thought applicable to Leith Hospital, "It can now truly be said that the two classes in this country who get the best treatment when suffering, are the very rich on the one hand and those on the other who could with difficulty if at all pay doctors' fees; because they are both treated on hospital principles, the rich because they can afford it, and the poor classes because the benevolent have provided it for them." Although these statements are somewhat self-congratulatory, appreciation from other sources is perhaps shown by the fact that in 1908 a request was made from the Imperial German Consulate in Leith that a commission from the city of Hamburg might be allowed to visit and inspect the hospital and study its function.[71]

In 1896 *"The Story of Leith Hospital"* from which many of the preceding quotations have been taken was published. This was a brief account of the hospital's history, its contemporary function and speculation about its future. It was compiled by members of the Board of Directors and staff but mainly by Mr Graham one of the directors. One of the comments on contemporary problems was, "The medical staff acknowledge with regret that they are compelled to refuse many deserving cases simply because there are no beds unoccupied. While this was the case with a remarkably mild, healthy winter, the effects would be vastly intensified by other atmospheric conditions or by any epidemic of sickness in town. Let it be particularly noted that the *Royal Infirmary cannot meet the deficiency*." This was part of an appeal for future support and a prediction that the future story of Leith Hospital would depend very much on Leith's own sons and daughters.

The year 1908 saw the establishment of an organisation which was to play an important part in the welfare of patients and staff during the hospital's existence and is still in being. Leith Hospital Samaritan Society of which more will be said later, was started by a group of ladies to provide needy patients with financial and other support which today is often statutorily provided. The Society's role in alleviating distress surrounding illness and admission to hospital is difficult to overstate.

In today's hospitals, lifts and telephones are essential features very much taken for granted. Estimates for a hydraulic lift were being obtained in 1889 the same year as the cost of connecting the hospital to a telephone system was being sought. This cost was £35 per annum but the advantages were not considered to be worth the expense![70] Four years later the hospital was connected to the telephone exchange but this time it was considered an unnecessary expense to connect the surgeons to the hospital by telephone![73]

It is possible to end the account of this period on an even lighter note. In November 1900 it was reported that patients were being disturbed at night by the noise of people leaving nearby premises. It would be natural to assume that these were one of the many places of entertainment or refreshment in Leith at that time. It comes as a surprise to learn that they were the Sheriff Brae Temperance Hall!

TABLE 2

Inpatient and Outpatient Statistics 1891, 1896 and 1906

	1891 (Before Closure) of Fever House	1896 (After Closure) of Fever House	1906 (After Opening) of New Pavilion
Inpatients			
Surgical	308	477	747
Medical	418	431	598
Fever	157	—	—
Gynaecological	—	85	141
Ophthalmic	—	30	38
	883	1023	1524
Operations	*	*	546
Outpatients (New patients only)			
Total	8932	11774	20893‡
Medical	*	*	4577
Surgical	*	*	5612
Gynaecological	*	176	495
Ophthalmic	*	910	1429
Teeth (extracted)	*	2373	1866
Electrical Department	—	—	13
Vaccinations	151	807	—
Cases Treated at home	4099	4731	6402
Seen by District Nurse	232	334	291†

*   not detailed.
‡   in 1906 a total of 30,704 return patients were seen.
†   4,562 visits were made.

TABLE 3

Classification of Disease and Infections: Inpatients 1906

MEDICAL WARD

General diseases	100
Poisoning	14
Skin	9
Circulatory system	89
Lymphatic system	10
Digestive system	62
Respiratory system	145
Urinary system	39
Nervous system	95

SURGICAL WARDS

General diseases	14
Nervous system	14
Circulatory system	11
Respiratory system	15
Lymphatic system	34
Digestive system	180
Genito. Urinary	62
Bones and Joints	60
Skin and cellular tissue	98
Malformations	24
Ears	4
Miscellaneous	9
Injuries	176
Burns	16

REFERENCES

CHAPTER 4

1. *Edinburgh & Leith Observer*, 22.12.1928.
2. Leith Hospital Annual Report, 1890.
3. *Medical Press.* 13.5.1891. p. 488.
4. Memorandum by Secretary, Leith Hospital Board of Directors, November 1890.
5. Leith Hospital Board of Directors, Minutes 16.9.1892.
6. Report from Leith Town Clerk's Office, 1894.
7. Marshall, J. S. Op. cit. p. 19.
8. Leith Hospital Annual Report, 1893.
9. Ibid., 1896.
10. Leith Hospital Board of Directors, Minutes 27.2.1893.
11. Ibid., 20.7.1893.
12. Leith Hospital Annual Report, 1893.
13. Leith Hospital Board of Directors, Minutes 9.12.1896.

14. Ibid., 29.4.1897.
15. Ibid., 13.5.1897.
16. Marshall, J. S. Op. cit. p. 24.
17. Leith Hospital Board of Directors, Minutes 15.1.1903.
18. Ibid., 17.7. 1901.
19. Marshall, J. S. Op. cit. p. 26.
20. Leith Hospital Annual Reports 1896, 1906.
21. Ibid., 1891.
22. Ibid., 1894.
23. Leith Hospital Board of Directors, Minutes 23.1.1901.
24. Leith Hospital Annual Report, 1908.
25. Ibid., 1910.
26. Ibid., 1907.
27. Leith Hospital Board of Directors, Minutes 16.11.1905.
28. Ibid., 26.3.1903.
29. Ibid., 17.2.1903.
30. Comrie, J. D. Op. cit. p. 616.
31. *Edinburgh Medical Journal*, (1903). Vol. 4, N.S. p. 287.
32. Craig, W. S. *History of the Royal College of Physicians of Edinburgh* (1976). p. 492. Edinburgh: Blackwell Scientific Publications.
33. *Edinburgh Medical Journal*, (1910). Vol. 5. N.S. p. 62.
34. Comrie, J. D. Op. cit. p. 700.
35. *Edinburgh Medical Journal*, (1911). Vol. 7, N.S. p. 64.
36. *Medical Directory*, 1906.
37. Anderson's College Dispensary, Glasgow. 5th Annual Report, 1883.
38. *Edinburgh Medical Journal*, (1931). Vol. 38, N.S. p. 545.
39. Leith Hospital Board of Directors, Minutes 17.3.1898.
40. *British Medical Journal*, (1946). Vol. 2 p. 443.
41. Ross, J. A. Op. cit. p. 91.
42. Ibid., p. 96.
43. *British Medical Journal*, (1930). Vol. 1. p. 1155.
44. Leith Hospital Board of Directors, Minutes 12.6.1895.
45. *Edinburgh Almanac* 1892, 1893.
46. *British Medical Journal*, (1938). Vol. 1. p. 260.
47. Ross, J. A. Op. cit. p. 200.
48. Comrie, J. D. Op. cit. p. 689.
49. Craig, W. S. Op. cit. p. 131.
50. *British Medical Journal*, (1924). Vol. 2. p. 836.
51. Sturrock, J. W. M. F. Shaw Memorial Lecture 1969.
52.. Leith Hospital Board of Directors, Minutes 20.6.1901.
53. Ibid., 9.4.1891.
54. *Edinburgh Evening News* 9.3.1896.
55. *Evening Dispatch* 10.3.1896.
56. Leith Hospital Board of Directors, Minutes 13.12.1895.
57. Ibid., 20.3.1890.
58. Ibid., 25.1.1891.
59. Ibid., 14.6.1894.
60. Ibid., 12.10.1899.
61. Ibid., 13.10.1898.
62. Ibid., 18.7.1907.

63.   Ibid., 18.10.1907.
64.   Ibid., 8.11.1900.
65.   Leith Hospital Board of Directors, Minutes 28.7.1904.
66.   Ibid., 26.5.1892.
67.   Ibid., 21.2.1895.
68.   Board of Directors and Staff. *The Story of Leith Hospital* 1896. pp. 26-38.
69.   Leith Hospital Board of Managers, Minutes 14.6.1909.
70.   Leith Hospital Annual Report, 1910.
71.   Leith Hospital Board of Managers, Minutes 16.7.1908.
72.   Ibid., 17.5.89.
73.   Ibid., 21.9.93.

War and Its Effects. 1911-1930

By 1911 Leith was the seventh largest town in Scotland with 80,000 inhabitants[1] many of whom were now wealthy ship owners and merchants but as James Scott Marshall points out the conditions of citizens at the opposite end of the social spectrum were very poor. Without sickness benefits, unemployment relief or old age pensions, working class families especially children suffered. He records that in 1906 an inquiry carried out by Leith School Board found that many children in Leith schools were not just malnourished, but starving.[2]

Fortunately for Leith Hospital many of the wealthy people of Leith were generous in their support of charitable activities and general support for the hospital became more popular. The onset of the 1914-18 war saw at least temporary improvement in unemployment but faced the hospital with many difficulties. The end of the war saw re-emergence of the issue of amalgamation of Leith with Edinburgh and indeed this took place in 1920 with inevitable effects on the community and the services within it. Post war economic depression also had its effects on charitable institutions.

The Impact of War

It was clear to many for a considerable time before its onset that war was approaching and that preparations should be made. In December 1913 the managers met with Fleet Surgeon Cooper to discuss arrangements for the admission in time of war of wounded men from mine sweepers and destroyers in the Firth of Forth.[3] Ten beds were offered with payment agreed at 3/6d. per day per patient. This figure was in line with that to be charged by Edinburgh Royal Infirmary but later when the British Hospitals Association suggested that a uniform charge be made throughout the United Kingdom, the managers of Leith Hospital expressed their view that voluntary hospitals were in different circumstances and that such an arrangement would not be equitable.[4] With the onset of war the number of beds first made available for naval casualties was thirty which rapidly increased to fifty to include military as well as naval personnel. To enable this commitment to be met Leith Town Council Public Health Committee provided fifty beds from East Pilton Hospital.[5] In the first few months of the war to the end of 1914, eighty-six soldiers and sailors were treated.[6] The bed complement of the hospital was in effect raised to 158 and this was done by "crowding up every corner"[7] and utilising the Winter Garden when necessary.

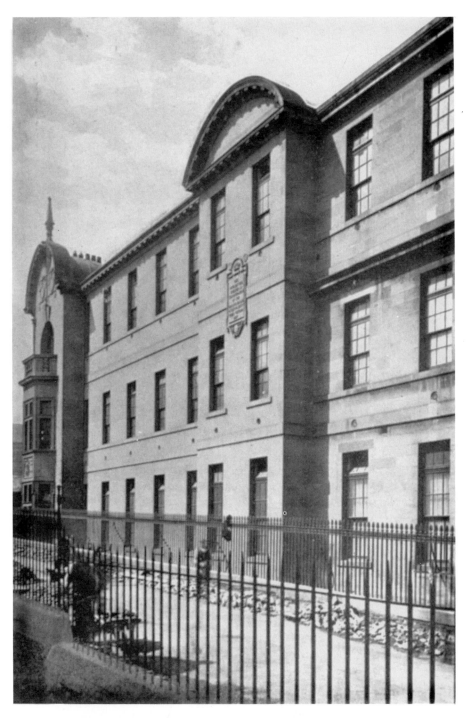

PLATE 5. Leith Hospital. Frontage of the new Jubilee Surgical Wing 1897

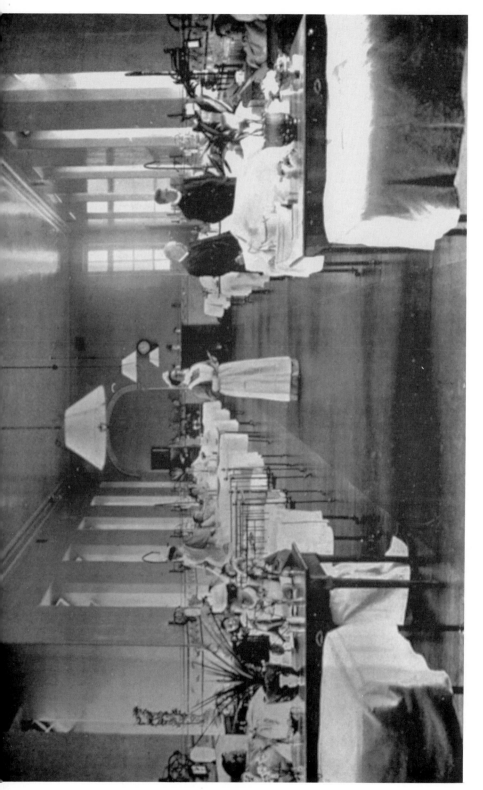

PLATE 6. Female surgical ward, circa 1900

The obvious increase in workload was accompanied by staffing difficulties. Doctors, nurses and other members of staff were keen to meet their service commitments and to volunteer for service with the armed forces. By December 1914 only one fully qualified resident medical officer remained in the hospital[8] and in 1917 the only qualified resident was appointed as medical officer to Leith War Hospital at Seafield; it was hoped that the advertisement for a person to fill this post might catch the eye of a retired doctor.[9] In the same year the Scottish Medical Service Emergency Committee expressed the need for more doctors in the army while recognising the depleted state of medical staff in hospitals in the city of Edinburgh and neighbourhood; it also appealed to hospitals to set at liberty for military service every available nurse.[10] The Lady Superintendent of Leith Hospital complained however that as a general rule, as soon as a nurse obtained her certificate, she went off voluntarily on military service.[11] Many served with great distinction and some of course with ultimate sacrifice. It is recorded with pride in the minutes of the Board of Managers in 1915 that the award of the Distinguished Service Order had been made to Captain A. G. A. Menzies, R.A.M.C. who had recently been a resident physician at the hospital.[12] Senior staff, physicians, surgeons and assistant physicians and surgeons also left for military service; Mr Wade, Mr Wilkie, Mr Scott Skirving, Mr Pirie Watson, Dr Ninian Bruce, Dr Torrance Thomson, Dr Mathewson, Dr Watson Wemyss, Dr Murray Wood, Dr Coombe and Mr Carlow, registrar, all left at different times and for varying periods. Mr J. W. Struthers on his return from military service was towards the end of 1918 the only surgeon working in the hospital at that time.[13] This great diminution of hospital staff would not have been compatible with adequate function of the hospital had not retired people rallied round; Dr Elder one of the consulting physicians and Mr Stewart one of the consulting surgeons were two former members of staff who helped in this way.[14] At other times staff from other hospitals helped out including Mr Quarry Wood and Mr Frank Jardine from the Edinburgh Royal Infirmary.[15]

Inevitably however there was disruption of services to the people of Leith. At one time in 1915 it was decided that no further patients could be admitted except soldiers and sailors — a circumstance which happily did not last long. At the same time outpatient clinics were reduced; all ophthalmic patients were referred to the Edinburgh Royal Infirmary from 1916[16] and the ear, nose and throat clinic was curtailed and stopped for a time but reopened by February 1918. As might be expected support from the community was unstinted, from the collection of medicine bottles for the hospital by Boy Scouts[17] to the untiring efforts of the Samaritan Society. Just as understandably there was a great desire to return to normality. Hardly a month after the armistice the managers were making application for the return of medical officers to their civilian duties[18] and by February 1919 they were requesting the appropriate departments to relieve the hospital of treating soldiers and repatriated prisoners.[19] Shortly after, all military patients had been transferred elsewhere.

The Changing Work of The Hospital

The war years saw some temporary retrenchment of services but the 1920s were years of vigorous growth. Curiously, although it is stated that "considerable numbers"[20] of wounded and disabled soldiers and sailors were treated during each of the war years, the hospital statistics do not differentiate between them and civilians so that precise numbers are unrecorded. Figures for inpatient and outpatient work in 1916 and 1926 are given in Table 4. Total inpatients treated in 1916 were 1354, a reduction compared with 1906 and which must have represented a very significant drop in civilians admitted. 1926 saw 1619 inpatients treated which did not include 436 children in the newly opened Children's Wing. Outpatient figures show a vast increase in activity by 1926 with 17,065 new patients treated and a total of 77,285 patients seen in all departments.

The institution was now functioning as an acute general hospital to a distinct community and capable of meeting the diagnostic and therapeutic needs of most patients presenting to it. A glance at a page of the operation book for 1912 gives some idea of the range of operations carried out (Table 5) and in addition an idea of the eminence of the staff involved at that time. At least two, Sir Henry Wade and Sir David Wilkie, became internationally renowned in the field of surgery.

The propriety of and necessity for treating some patients still exercised the thoughts of the Board. Cases of attempted suicide were, it was agreed, to be admitted to Edinburgh Royal Infirmary after consultation with the Chief Constable — a reflection of the laws in relation to suicide at that time.[21] On the other hand tuberculosis, other than pulmonary, continued to be treated as the Local Government Board could then provide sanitorium treatment for respiratory cases only.[22] During the war no cases of venereal disease were admitted as Edinburgh Royal Infirmary undertook the treatment of all such cases from Edinburgh, Leith and the Lothians,[23] although later in 1920 two rooms were allocated in the outpatient department for the running of a V.D. clinic one afternoon and one evening a week by the Medical Officer of Health.[24] Patients resident outwith Leith began to seek admission to the hospital, a matter which concerned the managers who felt that the number of such cases should be reduced as far as practicable.[25] The treatment of children was also a troublesome matter. By 1915 it was impossible to obtain medical practitioners to attend to necessitous children in the outpatient department[26] and it was agreed that a Dr Mowat acting in conjunction with the local Public Health Department could prescribe medicines for under school age children not otherwise provided for and that their prescriptions would be dispensed by the hospital. The following year accommodation was provided in the hospital for a clinic for pre-school children to be run by the Public Health Authorities[27] and in 1918 a request by the Medical Officer of Health that tonsillectomies on under fives be carried out was agreed to at a cost of £1 per case and they were carried out by Dr Douglas Guthrie.[28] In 1919 the Local Authority Child Welfare Clinic was discontinued at the hospital and moved elsewhere.[29]

The year 1918 in addition to seeing the end of the war saw the great worldwide pandemic of influenza which Leith did not of course escape. Cases first occurred in the community in July, abated after six weeks but returned in October. The hospital admitted eighty-six cases with complications of which ten died within forty-eight hours and fourteen later, a mortality rate of 27 per cent.[30]

One service which had been a keystone of the original hospital was to cease in this period. The attendance on patients in their own homes by a doctor resident in the hospital was a matter which had been debated for some time. One of the reasons for discontinuing this practice in January 1913 was financial, which will be referred to later, but in effect it was to break the remaining link with the old Leith Dispensary, as disposal of rescue equipment to the Local Authority broke the link with the Humane Society in 1885. From then on the hospital's outpatient commitment was the same as other hospitals.

Two further specialties were added to the medical scene in this time, anaesthetics in 1911 and otolaryngology in 1912. It has already been related how nurses received instruction in massage treatment of some patients in 1900. The beginnings of skilled physiotherapy appeared in 1915 when a certified masseuse requested permission to attend patients in hospital in the presence of her students.[32] This was granted and the progress towards establishment of a proper massage or physiotherapy department was made in 1921 when Miss Hastings, Director of the Edinburgh School of Massage, Medical Gymnastics and Medical Electricity expressed the wish to extend the massage work of the hospital by including Swedish remedial exercises. All necessary apparatus was supplied by the school and was under the charge of Miss C. D. Ewart.[33] These activities took place at first in the Winter Garden and later in the outpatient department. In 1926 it was decided that cases sent to the hospital for massage only should be under the supervision of the junior house surgeon.[34] The already established x-ray department had a difficult period just before and during the war; Dr Kerr, medical electrician had had to resign because of pressure of work and for some time x-ray photographs were taken at the hospital by Mr Williamson the dispenser who had some appropriate training.[35] In 1916 Dr Spence attended two days per week with the dispenser acting as his assistant until he (Dr Spence) was appointed radiographer (radiologist in modern terms) in 1918.[36]

Some indication of the clinical work undertaken during this time is given by the requests made by clinical staff for equipment and materials. In May 1923 authorisation was given by the House Committee for the use of insulin in one case in Dr Murray Woods ward.[37] As Banting and Best's paper on insulin did not appear until 1922 and related to animal experiments, this must have been one of the very early instances of its clinical use in Edinburgh. Indeed it was not until later that year that the first six cases treated in the Royal Infirmary of Edinburgh were reported in the Edinburgh Medical Journal.[38] They were treated "early in 1923" possibly as early as January.[39]

Later that decade requests were being made for ultraviolet light apparatus,[40] for a cystoscope (this had to be purchased from a New York firm at a cost of $125), for electrocautery apparatus[41] and a supply of radium.[42]

Although simple haematological and biochemical tests were carried out in the side rooms of the hospital by junior hospital staff it was becoming recognised that more specialised laboratory work was increasingly necessary in the diagnosis and management of patients. The obstetricians were requesting that the hospital defray the cost of Ascheim-Zondek pregnancy tests[43] and regular use was being made of the laboratory of the Royal College of Physicians of Edinburgh in Forrest Road, a facility which was appreciated for many years in the 20s, 30s and 40s and for which the hospital made a contribution of £50 per annum.[44] This laboratory, established by the College in 1887, was primarily for the prosecution of original research and was available to Fellows and Members of the College and later to Fellows of the Royal College of Surgeons of Edinburgh. It also undertook work for public bodies such as the Department of Health for Scotland and the Health Section of the League of Nations and for physicians and surgeons in their hospital practice; 15,176 specimens were sent for report in 1931. Several doctors working at Leith Hospital made use of the laboratory in their research and in investigational work and papers reporting this work were published by D. Berry Hart, William Fordyce, Henry Wade, David Wilkie, J. S. Fraser, J. K. Milne Dickie and Theodore Shennan.[45]

Finance and Administration

A few years before the onset of the war concern was being expressed about the implications of imminent social legislation on the funding of voluntary hospitals. The President of the Board of Managers, Mr Berry, speaking in 1911 was sceptical. "I do not understand the workings of Mr Lloyd George's mind," he averred but hoped that he (Lloyd George) had some idea that he was putting the working classes into a position of contributing more to charities in which they alone received the benefits.[46] The workings of Mr Lloyd George's mind were embodied in the National Insurance Act of 1911 whereby insurance against sickness and unemployment was to be paid for by contributions from the state, the employer and employee. Accordingly, a drop in subscriptions and donations to the hospital was expected. The following year the treasurer reported a serious falling off in subscriptions which he ascribed to "the malign influence of this terrible insurance act bogy",[47] and in 1913 he reported a further 10 per cent drop in contributions. Although he thought the prolonged dock strike in Leith had some bearing he had no doubt that the main cause was the insurance act and recounted how people collecting for the hospital had been told on several occasions "You had better apply to the Chancellor of the Exchequer Mr Lloyd George".[48]

Economic measures were inevitably sought and the ending of visiting patients in their own homes already referred to was certainly one. Moreover it was resolved that applicants for treatment in the outpatient department should be examined by a member of the honorary staff and if they were insured persons they should be referred to one of the doctors provided under the Act. It was further agreed that there would be no charge for inpatient care but insured persons would be admitted only as emergencies. If patients were admitted who were entitled to compensation under the Workmen's Compensation Act or to sick benefit under the National Insurance Act they were to arrange with the Lady Superintendent to give a contribution to funds.[49]

After the war economic measures and ways of increasing revenue was still concerning the administrators and in 1920 an "Economy Committee" was appointed. The following year it was recommended that a uniform charge be made in respect of the following; sixpence for each prescription dispensed, twopence for each dressing and sixpence for each massage or remedial exercise treatment.[50] Patients living outside Leith and who were in a position to pay would be charged two guineas per week as an inpatient. Later, in 1922 a uniform charge of 10/- for adults and 5/- for children was made for x-ray examinations.[51]

Despite all difficulties and with deficits in the ordinary income and expenditure account (£2,404 in 1912 and £2,341 in 1926) extraordinary income which included legacies, donations and endowments was well maintained and amounted to £15,579 in 1916[52] and £28,067 in 1927.[53] Total funds at the end of 1927 were £99,926 a sum which had been greatly boosted by the response to the War Memorial Appeal.

Considerable thought and organisation were now being used to augment funds. Before the war the Hospital Demonstration Committee planned processions and then flag days to raise money.[54] A new Leith Hospital Fund Committee was formed in 1927[55] and constituted in 1928 comprising representatives of the Friendly Societies, Trades Organisations and voluntary workers with a direct representation from the hospital managers. It continued this work, organising an annual pageant which became a feature of the life of the town and community. In 1929 this body raised £2,583 , collected, it was stressed, from mainly poor people in the town and calculated to represent a contribution of

2/9d. per household or 9d. per person.[56] The following year £2,694 was raised from this source, 75 per cent of the sum being in copper coins which must have had its problems in handling sheer weight.[57]

Larger sums continued to come from other sources and the wealthier citizens of the town. At the end of the war £3,000 was allocated for specific purposes from the Scottish branch of the British Red Cross Society.[58] This sum was eventually put to equipping the new Children's Wing.[59] Mention has already been made of the generous provision of convalescent facilities for the hospital by Mrs Jessie Campbell Currie. On her death in 1919 she bequeathed the home to the hospital and her sons and daughters continued the tradition of wealthy individual and family support by giving £5,000 to provide a fund for its maintenance.[60] Another enthusiastic beneficiary of the hospital (who also served on the Board of Directors and became Vice President) was Mr Thomas Cowan, a Leith ship owner. He donated over £23,000 to the hospital over a period of years including a sum of £10,000 in 1923 which was to be used in the reconstruction of the outpatient department.[61] His name is perpetuated in the "Cowan Hall" which became an important concourse and waiting area of the hospital and in which a medallion of the benefactor hangs.

The custom of donating money (£1,500 was sufficient) to endow beds was established by the end of the century and became a popular way of commemorating individuals, bodies and events to the extent that it provided a small historical mirror of the times and the community. Monarchs and their coronations, important local features like the docks and the death in battle of its young men were marked by brass plates on ward walls. Such a one is that in memory of Lieutenant Commander Mungo Campbell Gibson killed in action at the Dardanelles. [Plate 9]. That commemorating the rail disaster at Gretna in 1915 in which 200 officers and men of the seventh battalion The Royal Scots (recruited mainly from Leith) were killed, is a particularly poignant one and hung in ward one of the surgical block [plate 10].

The Board of Managers continued to function as it had following the incorporation of the hospital in 1907. In 1913 the Leith Medical Practitioners Association successfully requested that one of their number be appointed to represent it on the Board.[62] The Board had been from its inception an all male body. The first indication that this state of affairs was being questioned came in 1926 when a letter was received from the Edinburgh Society for Equal Citizenship asking that women be appointed to the Board.[63] The Board demurred and it was not until 1928 that the matter was raised again this time successfully when Mrs James Currie became the first woman manager.[64] Finally in this context, it is pleasing to record that Dr J. A. Gray was appointed a manager in 1922. He had been a medical officer of the hospital in the 1880s and 1890s and as medical officer of Health for Leith had not endeared himself to the hospital administration because of his outspoken concern for proper provision for infectious disease.[65] This was surely only appropriate recognition of his important contribution to medicine in Leith.

One interesting side issue which appeared in the minutes of the Board of Management in 1925 was the President's (ex Provost John Lindsay) suggestion that application should be made for a royal warrant so that the hospital could become the "Royal Leith Hospital". [66] Whether this suggestion received no support or application was made and rejected is not recorded.

The War Memorial and Children's Wing

The 1914-18 war was not long ended when thought was given by the town to the form of a suitable memorial to those who had died. The hospital formed a committee to further its own interests early in 1919[67] and later that year a committee to consider how the hospital was to develop in the post war years.[68] There was a clear desire to produce facilities for the treatment of children at Leith Hospital and money began to be donated to further a Children's Ward scheme. It was a most felicitous concept to combine this scheme with the erection of a War Memorial for Leith and the credit for it probably must be given to ex-Provost Lindsay, the last Provost of Leith before amalgamation with Edinburgh and a member of the Board of Managers of the hospital for many years. The community readily accepted this idea and plans for alterations and additions to the hospital were being considered by February 1920.[69] Money was eagerly contributed by the local population and some large sums donated including £20,000 from Mr John Hope, a former Leith business man then in London[70] and sums already mentioned from Mr Thomas Cowan. In 1922 Mr George Simpson, architect, produced plans for a building which was estimated to cost £25-30,000 and Colonel McIntosh of the Western Infirmary of Glasgow was appointed consulting architect.[71] In the event total costs came to around £40,000 but the financial response to the appeal had been so satisfactory that about £20,000 was kept as a nucleus of an endowment fund. Started in 1923 the new wing was formally opened in 1927 and was designed in stripped Tudor style [plate 11] and provided a ward for medical patients, a ward for surgical patients and four smaller wards, one for observation, one for eye patients and two for ear, nose and throat patients, a total of thirty-six beds or cots.[72] The hospital was now one of 141 beds and the general layout in relation to Mill Lane, King Street and Great Junction Street is shown in the sketch plan [plate 12]. The formal opening of the new wing was undertaken on 29th January 1927 by Sir John Gilmour, Secretary of State for Scotland, the front page of the official programme emphasising the dual nature of the building as war memorial and Children's Wing of a hospital [plate 13]. Later that year ex-Provost Lindsay as the then President of the Board of Managers and representing the war memorial committee formally handed over to the managers the copy of resolution adopted by the committee including; "(1) The Children's Wing and equipment thereof; (2) Addition to the nurses home and furniture therein; and (3) An endowment fund representing £31,600."[73]

As implied above alteration to the nurses home had been agreed to in 1925[74] and extensive alterations to the outpatient department made at the time of the construction of the Children's Wing. The only other building undertaken at this time was a chapel to facilitate burial services which was undertaken in 1925.[75]

As end pieces to the story of Leith's War Memorial and the Children's Wing of Leith Hospital it should be recorded that from a population in 1914 of 84,000 people, 14,200 Leithers enlisted of whom 2205 perished, their names being recorded in the role of honour which was entrusted to the managers of Leith Hospital. On the home front Leith had sustained a Zeppelin raid with loss of life and damage (but not to the hospital), the tragedy of the Gretna disaster, but more happily the repatriation of 40,000 prisoners of war through the port and ultimately the spectacle of the anchorage off the port of the surrendered German fleet.[76] Finally in 1930 the British Legion suggested that the annual wreath laying ceremony take place at the war memorial, that is just outside the entrance to the Children's Wing, instead of at the statue of Queen Victoria as before.[77] This was the beginning of a practice which has persisted to the present time.

Hospital Staffing

Little change took place with regard to numbers and function of staff during this time except that appropriate to the opening of the Children's Wing. Specialist paediatric physicians and surgeons were not at that time appointed. Instead some of the honorary physicians and surgeons already in post undertook duties in the Children's Wing. Dr Watson Wemyss assumed full charge of the children's medical ward relinquishing his six beds in the main hospital. Dr Mathewson assisted Dr Murray Wood and Dr W. A. Alexander assisted Dr Mathewson, and had charge of the children's medical ward in Dr Watson Wemyss's absence. Similarly Mr Shaw took charge of the children's surgical ward also giving up his beds in the main hospital. Mr Mitchell assisted Mr Carlow and had charge of the children's surgical ward in Mr Shaw's absence. The staffing difficulties during the war were resolved after 1918, the junior medical and surgical posts continuing to be popular with recent graduates. There was a gap in the 1920s in the appointment of an anaesthetist to the hospital but senior surgical staff considered that anaesthetising could be done by resident staff with the aid of specialist anaesthetists called in difficult cases.[78] In 1927 the question of residents' remuneration or honorarium was discussed and it was recommended that the war time measure of payment be discontinued and that in future appointments should be made, as it was euphemistically put, "without pecuniary consideration".[79]

Dr William Elder on relinquishing his post as physician was appointed a consulting physician in 1910 and remained so until his death in 1931. Similarly Dr Langwill became a consulting physician from 1912 until 1946. Appointed consulting physician in 1921 Dr Edwin Matthew had also served Leith Hospital as a physician.

Edwin Matthew (1870-1950). He graduated MA from Aberdeen University in 1889 and was a member of the teaching profession until he decided to study medicine graduating MB at Edinburgh in 1897 and being awarded the Ettles prize as outstanding student. Fellowship of the Royal College of Physicians of Edinburgh came in 1906 and two years later he was awarded the gold medal for his MD thesis on "Vaso dilator substances in high blood pressure". In addition to becoming physician to Leith Hospital from 1912-1921 he was physician to the Royal Dispensary and then to the Royal Infirmary. The excellence of his clinical skills and well renowned teaching ability were recognised in his appointment to the Moncrief Arnott Chair of Clinical Medicine at Edinburgh University.[80]

Other physicians appointed in this time were John Easson, A. Murray Wood, G. D. Mathewson and H. L. Watson Wemyss.

John Easson (1874-1964). After graduating MB with first class honours at Edinburgh and being awarded the gold medal for his MD thesis in 1905 he studied at Heidelberg. He became a Fellow of the Royal College of Physicians of Edinburgh in 1902. Following his early association with Leith Hospital he joined the Honorary staff of Edinburgh Royal Infirmary. During the First World War he served as a Major RAMC with the 58th Scottish General Hospital. He retired from the Royal Infirmary in 1938 but in 1940 was invited to assume charge of medical wards at Chalmers Hospital where he remained until 1950. Endocrinology interested him particularly and his monograph "Exophthalmic Goitre" published in 1927 was well received.[81]

Arthur Murray Wood (1878-1945). Graduating with first class honours at Edinburgh in 1900 he subsequently graduated MD, obtained the Diploma of Public Health and Fellowship of the Royal College of Physicians of Edinburgh. Before the 1914-18 war he was in general practice in Leith and assistant medical officer to Leith Hospital. As a major in the RAMC he stayed with the hospital he commanded when it was overrun by the Germans and was thanked in person by the Kaiser for his devotion to duty. He was the first officer ashore from the ship which repatriated prisoners of war at Leith. He later became physician to Leith Hospital and was appointed consulting physician in 1931 but served the hospital devotedly in the Second World War. His son, Dr A. E. S. Wood also served the community of Leith as general practitioner for many years.[82]

George Douglas Mathewson (1883-1936). He graduated in Edinburgh in 1905 and became a Fellow of the Royal College of Physicians of Edinburgh in 1912. Before becoming Physician to Leith Hospital he was assistant to the Professor of Medicine and clinical tutor at Edinburgh Royal Infirmary later returning there as Physician. He had a special interest in diseases of the heart and published numerous articles on this topic as well as writing "The Examination of the Heart by Graphic Methods" in the second edition of the *Encyclopaedia Medica.*

Herbert Lindesay Watson Wemyss (1885-1933). The son of a general practitioner near Dundee and grandson of a former surgeon to Edinburgh Royal Infirmary he graduated in 1908, took his M.D. in 1910 and became a Fellow of the Royal College of Physicians of Edinburgh in 1914. Before the war he studied in Berlin and during the war was Medical Officer to the Red Cross Hospital in Dalmeny House, later serving in Malta. As well as being physician to Leith Hospital he was a physician to the Royal Dispensary, to the Deaconess Hospital and the Edinburgh Royal Infirmary. He was Secretary of the Harveian Society for many years.[84]

Some physicians who achieved eminence were assistant medical officers at Leith for relatively short periods. Such were David Halliday Croom (from 1910-1919), son of the former Professor of Obstetrics at Edinburgh and father of the future President of the Royal College of Physicians of Edinburgh; W. D. D. Small (from 1923-1925) a future Consultant to the army in the Middle East and President of the Royal College of Physicians of Edinburgh; W. A. Alexander (from 1926-1929) eventually to become physician to the Edinburgh Royal Infirmary and another President of the Royal College of Physicians of Edinburgh; A. R. Gilchrist (for a very short time), cardiologist and future president of the Royal College of Physicians of Edinburgh; and finally L. S. P. (Sir Stanley) Davidson who became Professor of Medicine at Edinburgh, a renowned haematologist and a President of the Royal College of Physicians of Edinburgh and who records his position as assistant physician to Leith Hospital on the title page of his important book with G. L. Gulland on *"Pernicious Anaemia"* [plate 14].

The surgical services of the hospital were also run by men of distinction during this time, the three consulting surgeons being J. W. Struthers, Henry Wade and D. P. D. Wilkie. It gives pleasure to record all three had close connections with the hospital as surgeons or assistant surgeons before their appointment as consulting surgeons.

John William ("Jock") Struthers (1874-1953) was a son of Sir John Struthers, former President of the Board of Directors of Leith Hospital, and therefore a nephew of Dr James Struthers who had been a medical officer and consulting physician to Leith Hospital. He served as surgeon to Leith Hospital from 1911 to 1925 and subsequently as surgeon to Edinburgh Royal Infirmary. Particularly interested in disorders of the bone he made original contributions on the elucidation of the pathology and treatment of generalised osteitis fibrosa. He was President of the Royal College of Surgeons of Edinburgh from 1941-1943.[85]

Sir Henry Wade CMG, DSO (1877-1955). Wade served Leith Hospital as assistant surgeon from 1909-1919, as surgeon from 1920-1926 and was appointed consulting surgeon from 1927 until his death. His achievements and distinctions are legend. An honours MB graduate of 1898, he served in the South African war and became a Fellow of the Royal College of Surgeons of Edinburgh in 1903 and was awarded the gold medal for his MD thesis. He had a further impressive career in the First World War becoming consulting surgeon to the Egyptian Expeditionary Force and being awarded the Distinguished Service Order. Between the wars he achieved a world reputation in urology and although he retired from his post as surgeon to Edinburgh Royal Infirmary in 1939, with the onset of the Second World War he was appointed a consulting surgeon at Bangour Emergency Medical Service Hospital remaining in active surgical practice for the next five years.[86]

Sir David Percival Dalbreck Wilkie, OBE (1882-1938) was assistant surgeon at Leith Hospital from 1911 to 1924 and consulting surgeon from then until his death. A native of Kirriemuir and a friend of J. M. Barrie, he became internationally known as a surgeon particularly for his abdominal surgery and as a researcher and teacher. Graduating MD and ChM he became a Fellow of the Royal College of Surgeons of Edinburgh and also of the Royal College of Surgeons in England. His early career was interrupted by service in the Royal Naval Volunteer Reserve in the 1914-18 war when he served in hospital ships in the Mediterranean. His skills as a teacher and researcher were reason for his appointment to the Chair of Systematic Surgery at Edinburgh and surgeon to the Royal Infirmary of Edinburgh. The research laboratory which he founded became after his death the Wilkie Research Laboratory. He was knighted in 1936 before his comparatively early death at fifty-six and was the recipient of many honours from the United Kingdom and overseas.[87]

The surgeons appointed during this time were A. Pirrie Watson, W. W. Carlow and J. J. M. Shaw.

Alexander Pirrie Watson, OBE (military) (1880-1943) was surgeon to Leith Hospital for thirteen years between 1925 and 1938 and was pathologist and assistant surgeon before this. An Aberdonian and ChM gold medalist he was a territorial army officer and as medical officer to the 4th Battalion Royal Scots, served at Gallipoli and then Egypt and Palestine. After the war he continued his interest in the territorial army and eventually became Colonel and ADMS of the 52nd (Lowland) Division. He became surgeon in charge of wards at the Edinburgh Royal Infirmary in 1937.[88]

Walter Waddell Carlow (1885-1965) was a devoted servant of Leith Hospital. Graduating MB in 1910 he became a Fellow of the Royal College of Surgeons in 1912. He was appointed registrar to the hospital in

1914 but served in the First World War in Salonika. After a period as assistant surgeon he became surgeon at Leith Hospital in 1926 and served until his retirement carrying an immense burden of emergency surgery during the Second World War when many of his younger colleagues were on war service. He was an excellent practical surgeon having an aptitude for engineering and was adept at orthopaedics.[89]

John James McIntosh Shaw, MC (1886-1940), was the founder of plastic surgery in Edinburgh. Having had a distinguished record in the First World War in France he worked on injuries to the face and jaw in The Queen's Hospital Sidcup for several years before returning to be appointed to the staff of Leith Hospital and the Edinburgh Royal Infirmary in 1927. He continued his work on plastic surgery but was primarily a general surgeon. In 1939 he became Colonel and Consulting Surgeon to the army in the Middle East but died at the age of fifty-four of acute bacillary dysentery.[90]

Mention should also be made of the appointment as assistant surgeon to Leith Hospital from 1925-1930 of Mr (later Sir) Walter Mercer, later to become the first Professor of Orthopaedics at Edinburgh University, and R. Leslie Stewart, assistant surgeon from 1927.

The gynaecologists appointed during this time were William Fordyce, J. Lamond Lackey and W. F. T. Haultain.

William Fordyce (1863-1941), was gynaecologist to Leith Hospital from 1911-1923 and later obstetrician to Simpson Memorial Hospital and gynaecologist to Edinburgh Royal Infirmary. Graduating MB at Edinburgh in 1888 with first class honours he was one of the original Fellows of the new Royal College of Obstetricians and Gynaecologists in 1929. He was renowned for his prowess as an after dinner speaker and wrote verse which he had printed privately in a volume entitled *"The Old Sport and Other Verses"*. He was appointed the consulting gynaecologist to Leith Hospital in 1923.[91]

James Lamond Lackie (1867-1924), graduated in 1889 at Edinburgh with first class honours. He took his MD in 1894 and became a Fellow of the Royal College of Physicians of Edinburgh in 1896. He undertook general practice in England for some time but on returning north started a career in obstetrics and gynaecology by becoming assistant to Dr (Sir) J. H. Croom. He was gynaecologist to Leith Hospital for only two years between 1922 and 1924 but was also on the staff of the Edinburgh Maternity Hospital and the Edinburgh Hospital for Diseases of Women.[92]

William Francis Theodore Haultain, OBE, MC (1893-1958). Appointed to Leith Hospital to replace Lamond Lackey he served as gynaecologist from 1925-1932 and was then appointed consulting gynaecologist. He was studying medicine at Cambridge in 1914 when he joined the Red Cross but was sent back to Edinburgh to continue his medical studies which he did graduating in 1916. He served with distinction in the RAMC from then until 1919 in France and Palestine and rose to the rank of lieutenant colonel. He became a Fellow of the Royal College of Surgeons of Edinburgh in 1922, a Fellow of the Royal College of Obstetricians and Gynaecologists in 1954 and a Fellow of the Royal College of Physicians of Edinburgh in 1945. After a consultant post in Edinburgh Royal Infirmary he retired in 1947 but in 1948 and the start of the National Health Service he took charge of wards at Bangour Hospital and the Eastern General Hospital, Edinburgh until shortly before his death in 1958. With C. D. Kennedy he produced a well known textbook *"A Practical Handbook of Midwifery and Gynaecology"*.[93]

Douglas Millar was assistant gynaecologist from 1925-1928 and both Clifford Kennedy and E. Chalmers Fahmy became assistants in 1929.

Four ophthalmic surgeons were appointed in this time, H. M. Traquair, Ernest H. Cameron, C. W. Graham and Laura M. Ligertwood.

Harry Moss Traquair (1875-1954), was a member of Leith Hospital staff from 1912-1915. He is best known for the work which resulted in the publication in 1927 of his *"An Introduction to Clinical Perimetry"*, which is now a classic of medical literature. Later on the staff of Edinburgh Royal Infirmary he was known as an excellent clinical teacher.[94]

Ernest Hugh Cameron (1889-1983), served Leith Hospital from 1915-1925 with an interruption during the war years when he served in the RAMC in Salonika and Egypt. He had taken the Fellowship of the Royal College of Surgeons of Edinburgh in 1914. He left Leith Hospital to become assistant and then surgeon to the Ophthalmic Department of Edinburgh Royal Infirmary and was appointed consulting surgeon to Leith Hospital in 1932.[95]

Charles William Graham (1888-1978). Qualifying in 1911 and taking the Fellowship of the Royal College of Surgeons of Edinburgh in 1921 he spent six years as Admiralty Surgeon in Shetland in demanding surgical practice. On devoting himself to surgical ophthalmology he became a member of staff of Leith Hospital and then the Edinburgh Royal Infirmary. He served in the Middle East from 1940-42.[96]

The first four aural surgeons (ear, nose and throat specialists) to be appointed were John S. Fraser in 1912, J. K. Milne Dickie in 1915, W. T. Gardiner in 1920 and J. Ewart Martin in 1926. One of the assistant ENT surgeons, appointed in 1929, was I. Simson Hall.

John Smith Fraser (1874-1936). Graduating in Edinburgh in 1897 he was in general practice in Litchfield for five years before undertaking further study in London and Vienna and taking the Fellowship of the Royal College of Surgeons of Edinburgh in 1905. Devoting himself thereafter to his specialty he became surgeon to the E.N.T. Department at Edinburgh Royal Infirmary on leaving Leith Hospital. He wrote the section on Diseases of the Ear in Wrights *"Diseases of the Nose, Throat and Ear"*.[97]

George Ewart Martin (1889-1950). He qualified in 1913, worked as a surgical specialist in a Casualty Clearing Station in the 1st World War and was one of the first ENT specialists in the RAMC Becoming an FRCSE in 1920 he studied in Philadelphia under Chevalier Jackson. Later he became surgeon in charge, ENT Department, Edinburgh Royal Infirmary as well as at Leith, Bangour, Kirkcaldy and Kelso. He wrote the section on nasal sinuses in Logan Turner's textbook.[98]

The first record of the appointment of an anaesthetist was that of Dr H. Torrance Thomson in 1911 followed by Dr Sybil Rutherford in 1928. Dr J. W. L. Spence became radiologist in 1918 and held this post until 1931.

John W. L. Spence (1871-1930), was born in Smyrna and spent the first decade of his life in the near East. Graduating in Edinburgh in 1898 he went into practice in Newcastle but became interested in radiology after a chance meeting with Dr Röntgen. He became assistant to Dr Dawson Tait in the Edinburgh Royal Infirmary and then radiologist to Royal Hospital for Sick Children, Edinburgh, Leith Hospital and Deaconess Hospital. He was one of the early radiologists who suffered severe x-ray dermatitis and ulceration and underwent numerous amputations to upper limbs between 1907 and 1930.[99]

Pathologists continued to be appointed for short periods most of them combining the pathology work with surgical duties. They included J. H. H. Pirrie, A. Pirrie Watson, George Richardson, Andrew Rutherford, J. J. M. Shaw, R. Leslie Stewart and David Band.

The nursing services were for most of this time under the supervision of Miss J. K. MacLean who was Lady Superintendent from 1908-1929. Under her guidance the training of nurses progressed. A certificate of nursing[100] was in existence before the war as was a silver medal presented annually to the best nurse.[101] However, this practice must have lapsed probably during the war as medals were reintroduced in the 1930s as will be recorded later. Badges for nurses completing their training were introduced in 1924.[102] Lectures to nurses suffered because of lack of medical staff during the war;[103] for example no one was available to teach veneral diseases and application was made to the National Council for Combating Venereal Disease for a lecturer.[104] Although nursing training at the hospital was approved by the General Nursing Council in 1923 Miss MacLean advised the managers in 1924 that a tutor was required to supervise the programme of training[105] but no action appears to have been taken until she returned to the attack in 1926 when she warned the managers that none of the nurses from the hospital were entering the State Registration Examination. If they failed to do so, she pointed out, the hospital would in all probability be struck off the list of approved training centres. Faced with such a threat the managers resolved to appoint a sister tutor at once to allow nurses to receive the special tuition necessary.[106] In 1929 a certificated sister tutor was appointed at a salary of £150 per annum.[107] In 1926 a nursing link with the Edinburgh Hospital and Dispensary for Women (Bruntsfield

Hospital) was created when it was agreed to accept probationers from Bruntsfield to train at Leith provided they trained for three years and started at Leith Hospital.[108]

Nursing salaries seemed grievously low at that time. In 1916 the Lady Superintendent received £125 per annum plus board and apartment and by 1927 this had risen to £150 per annum.[109] Sisters, however, in 1916 received only between £34 and £42 per annum plus uniform, board and apartment, this by 1919 rising to £40-£50 (in 1919 the radiographer received £100 per annum and the dispenser £200 per annum but without of course other emoluments).[110] Probationers in 1918 received £12, £16 and £20 respectively in their first, second and third years plus of course board and apartments.[111] Although the professional status of nursing had risen gradually it still lagged far behind in remuneration.

TABLE 4

Inpatient and Outpatient Statistics 1916 and 1926

	1916		1926
Inpatients	ADULT	ADULT	PAEDIATRIC+
Surgical	776	734	142
Medical	437	495	189
Gynaecological	122	221	—
Ophthalmic	19	60	11
Ear, nose and throat	—	109	94
	1354	1619	436
Operations	552	819*	
Outpatients (New patients only)‡			
Surgical	5244		7050
Medical	2877		4647
Gynaecological	453		823
Ophthalmic	645		1593
Ear, nose and throat	153		1187
(Electrical Dept. total)	421		1152
Physiotherapy	—		615
	9352		17,065

+   not full year
*   Surgical 537
     Gynaecological 214
     Ophthalmic 28
     Ear, nose and throat 40
‡   In 1916 a total of 28,527 return patients were seen and in 1926, 60,230.

TABLE 5

Case Ref.	Date of Operation	Name	Age	Operation for	Anaes-thetic	Result	Remarks	Surgeon
127	March 23rd	—	30	Varicocele	C	Cure	Radical cure	Mr Wilkie
128	March 23rd	—	24	Osteomyelitis Femur	C	Improved	Satisfactory	Mr Wilkie
129	March 26th	—	43	Strangulated Hernia Femoral	C	Cure	Radical cure	Mr Skirving
130	March 30th	—	58	Carcinoma Pelvic Colon	C	Death	Colostomy	Mr Struthers
131	March 27th	—	22	Stenosed Cervix	C	Cure	Curetage Dilatation	Dr Lackie
132	March 29th	—	51	Prolapsed uterus	D	Death	Ant. Colporrhaphy & Perineor-raphy	Dr Lackie
133	March 29th	—	43	Menorrhagia	C	Cure	Curettage	Dr Lackie
134	March 29th	—	37	Carcinoma Cervix	C	I.S.Q.	Cervix Curetted & Cauterised	Dr Lackie
135	March 29th	—	22	Lacerated Hand	C	Improved	Fingers amputated (4)	Mr Wilkie
136	March 30th	—	73	Glands in neck	C	Improved	Excised	Mr Struthers
137	March 29th	—	2	Hypospadias	C	Improved	Plastic Op.	Mr Skirving
138	March 30th	—	64	Rodent ulcer	C	Improved	Skin grafted	Mr Struthers
139	March 26th	—	69	Malignant liver?	C	Death	Laparotomy	Mr Skirving
139a	March 27th	—	34	Displacement of semilunar L. Knee	C	Cure	Excision	Mr Skirving
140	April 4th	—	19	L. Ing. Hernia	C	Cure	Rad. cure	Mr Wade
141	April 5th	—	26	L. Ing. Hernia	C	Cure	Rad. cure	Mr Skirving
142	April 5th	—	2	Osteomyelitis of Femur	C	Cure	Trephined femur	Mr Skirving
143	April 5th	—	67	Old suprapubic cystotomy	C	Cure	Ext. urethrotomy suprapubic cystotomy	Mr Skirving
144	April 6th	—	9	Glands in neck	C	Cure	Excision of glands	Mr Struthers
145	April 6th	—	17	Glands in neck	C	Cure	Excision of glands	Mr Struthers
146	April 10th	—	15	Appendicitis	C	Cure	Appendicectomy	Mr Struthers
147	April 11th	—	32	Varicocele	C	Cure	Rad. cure	Mr Wade
148	April 11th	—	2	Supp. arthritis		Cure	Trephined through head of femur into joint	Mr Wade
149	April 11th	—	17	Glands in neck (R)		Cure	Excision of glands	Mr Wade
150	April 11th	—	21	Malunion of (R) Radius		Cure	Divided and set	Mr Wade
151	April 11th	—	40	Dislocation of (R) Shoulder		Improved	Excision head of humerus	Mr Wade
152	April 12th	—	15	Cold abscess		Improved	Opened and scraped	Mr Struthers
153	April 12th	—	2½	Hypospadias		Cure	Dorsal plastic op.	Mr Struthers

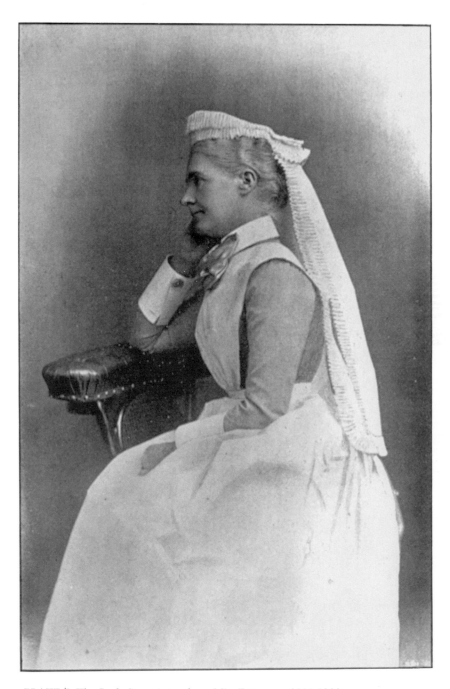

PLATE 7. The Lady Superintendent. Miss Paterson, 1892-1908

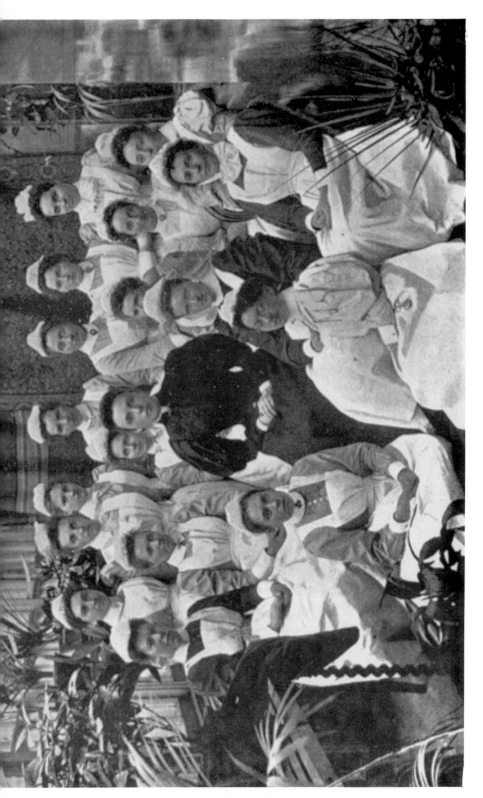

PLATE 8. A group of nurses, circa 1896

REFERENCES

CHAPTER 5

1.   Pryde, G., S. (1962). *A New History of Scotland*, Vol. 2, p. 258, Edinburgh; Thomas Nelson.
2.   Marshall, J. S. (1986) *The Life and Times of Leith.* p. 181, Edinburgh; James Donald.
3.   Leith Hospital Board of Managers, Minutes 18.12.1913.
4.   Ibid., 21.1.1915.
5.   Ibid., 12.11.1914.
6.   Leith Hospital Annual Report, 1914.
7.   Ibid., 1915.
8.   Leith Hospital Board of Managers, Minutes 10.12.1914.
9.   Ibid., 8.2.1917.
10.   Ibid., 10.5.1917.
11.   Ibid., 10.5.1917.
12.   Ibid., 18.11.1915.
13.   Ibid., 17.10.1918.
14.   Ibid., 10.12.1914.
15.   Ibid., 13.4.1917.
16.   Ibid., 20.7.1916.
17.   Ibid., 16.3.1916.
18.   Ibid., 19.12.1918.
19.   Ibid., 13.2.19   .
20.   Leith Hospital Annual Report 1916.
21.   Leith Hospital Board of Managers, Minutes 17.10.1912.
22.   Ibid., 19.12.1912.
23.   Ibid., 20.9.1917.
24.   Ibid., 12.2.1920.
25.   Ibid., 14.1.1915.
26.   Ibid., 13.5.1915.
27.   Ibid., 9.11.1916.
28.   Ibid., 21.2.1918.
29.   Ibid., 20.2.1919.
30.   Leith Hospital Annual Report 1918.
31.   Leith Hospital Board of Managers, Minutes 24.12.1912.
32.   Ibid., 14.10.1915.
33.   Ibid., 20.1.1921.
34.   Ibid., 18.11.1926.
35.   Leith Hospital Annual Report 1912.
36.   Leith Hospital Board of Managers, Minutes 1.5.1916.
37.   Ibid., 10.5.1923.
38.   Meakins, J. et al. *Edinburgh Medical Journal* (1923), Vol. 30, p. 127.
39.   Clarke, Dr Basil F., Personal Communication.
40.   Leith Hospital Board of Managers, Minutes 18.4.1929.
41.   Ibid., 13.6.1929.
42.   Ibid., 12.12.1929.
43.   Ibid., 20.6.1929.
44.   Ibid., 18.9.1928.

45.   Ritchie, J. (1953) *History of the Laboratory of the Royal College of Physicians of Edinburgh,* pp. 109-150.
46.   Leith Hospital Annual Report, 1911.
47.   Ibid., 1912.
48.   Ibid., 1913.
49.   Leith Hospital Board of Managers, Minutes 24.12.1912.
50.   Ibid., 14.10.1921.
51.   Ibid., 18.5.1922.
52.   Leith Hospital Annual Report 1916.
53.   Leith Hospital Annual Report 1927.
54.   Leith Hospital Board of Managers, Minutes 10.4.1915.
55.   Ibid., 10.2.1927.
56.   Ibid., 10.7.1929.
57.   Ibid., 18.9.1930.
58.   Ibid., 12.11.1919.
59.   Ibid., 16.9.1920.
60.   Leith Hospital Annual Report, 1919.
61.   Leith Hospital Board of Managers, Minutes 20.12.1923.
62.   Ibid., 16.1.1913.
63.   Ibid., 18.2.1926.
64.   Ibid., 16.2.1928.
65.   Leith Hospital Annual Report, 1922.
66.   Leith Hospital Board of Managers, Minutes 14.5.1925.
67.   Ibid., 20.2.1919.
68.   Ibid., 11.12.1919.
69.   Ibid., 19.2.1920.
70.   Marshall, J. S. (1978) *Leith's Greatest Charity,* p. 29.
71.   Leith Hospital Board of Managers, Minutes 24.2.1922.
72.   *Leith Observer,* 29.6.1927.
73.   Leith Hospital Board of Managers, Minutes 15.12.1927.
74.   Ibid., 21.3.1925.
75.   Ibid., 19.2.1925.
76.   *Leith Observer,* 29.6.1927.
77.   Leith Hospital Board of Managers, Minutes 9.10.1930.
78.   Ibid., 21.2.1924.
79.   Ibid., 14.7.1927.
80.   *Edinburgh Medical Journal* (1950), Vol. 57. p. 489.
81.   *British Medical Journal* (1964), Vol. 2. p. 1401.
82.   Wood, Dr A. E. S., Personal Communication.
83.   *British Medical Journal* (1936), Vol. 1. p. 91.
84.   *British Medical Journal* (1933), Vol. 1. p. 294.
85.   Ross, J. A. Op. cit. p. 109.
86.   Ibid., p. 78.
87.   Ibid., p. 123.
88.   Ibid., p. 115.
89.   *British Medical Journal* (1965), Vol. 2., p. 426.
90.   Ross, J. A. Op. cit. p. 73.
91.   Ibid., p. 216.
92.   *Edinburgh Medical Journal* (1924), Vol. 31, p. 104.
93.   *British Medical Journal* (1958), Vol. 2, p. 1359.

94.   Ross, J. A. Op. cit., p. 200.
95.   *British Medical Journal* (1983), Vol. 2, p. 1068.
96.   *British Medical Journal* (1978), Vol. 1, p. 1428.
97.   *British Medical Journal* (1936), Vol. 1, p. 1081.
98.   *British Medical Journal* (1950), Vol. 1, p. 848.
99.   *Edinburgh Medical Journal* (1930), Vol. 37, p. 312.
100.   Leith Hospital Board of Managers, Minutes 8.2.1912.
101.   Ibid., 9.3.1912.
102.   Ibid., 10.4.1924.
103.   Ibid., 18.11.1915.
104.   Ibid., 12.12.1918.
105.   Ibid., 9.10.1924.
106.   Ibid., 8.4.1926.
107.   Ibid., 29.11.1929.
108.   Ibid., 15.4.1926.
109.   Ibid., 19.5.1927.
110.   Ibid., 15.5.1919.
111.   Ibid., 14.11.1918.

The Apogee of the Voluntary Hospital
1931-1948

The hospital, like the community it served and the nation in general, slowly recovered from the effects of war, the general strike and economic depression before battening down once more against the storms of war. By the mid 1930s the voluntary hospital was probably at its peak as regards financial integrity and confidence for the future although the work accomplished continued to increase into the 1940s. Confidence became eroded however in the post war economic and political climate and with the increasing realisation that nationalisation of hospitals was to come about.

Hospital Activity Before the Second World War

Clinical Work

A glance at patient statistics for 1936[1] (Table 6) shows the steady increase in inpatient and outpatient work. 2725 adults and children were treated as inpatients in that year and a total of 18,276 new outpatients seen, return patients totalling almost 75,000. Most departments had increased their workload but the increase in paediatric activity, in E.N.T. work and the addition of a dermatology clinic were the main causes of the increase. The inpatient work was accomplished with a bed complement at that time of 151, the average number of patients resident daily being 131 and the cost per occupied bed per year amounting to £149 9/10d. The average stay of adult patients in hospital was twenty-nine days for medical patients, twenty-one days for surgical and an average for all wards of eighteen days. The average stay for children was fourteen days. Crude mortality figures for adult patients were 16.5 per cent for medical and 10.3 per cent for surgical; what is surprising is the 12.5 per cent mortality of paediatric medical patients and 3.7 per cent for surgical. Indeed comment had been made at a board meeting in 1933 about the number of deaths in the children's wing when it was explained by medical staff that many of the children dying had been admitted *in extremis*, in the last stages of their disease.[2]

Taking the month of January 1936, thirty-four patients were admitted to the medical wards half of whom had respiratory infections, cardiac disease or pernicious anaemia (no cerebrovascular disease!) and seven of the ten deaths were pneumonia or rheumatic heart disease.[3]

Sixty-four patients were admitted that same month to the surgical wards, thirty-seven of whom had appendicitis, infections or trauma and burns; of the six deaths four were trauma or burns.[4] In the children's medical ward twenty-seven of the thirty-four admissions were pneumonias or bronchitis of whom three died.[5] A total of 232 patients from hospital were accommodated in the convalescent home at Corstorphine that year and eighty-two children convalesced in the home at North Berwick.

By 1946[6] and after return to peacetime conditions, overall activity had again increased although there was fluctuation in some departments. The hospital in that year treated 3,344 inpatients and coped with an impressive grand total of 99,846 outpatient attendances as well as performing 1,729 operations on inpatients and 964 operations on outpatients.

Hidden within the framework of figures are of course a number of matters reflecting changes in medical and surgical practice as well as changes in the life of the community and society in general. For example the motor car began to contribute significantly to the pattern of trauma and in 1931 the managers decided that in view of the provisions within the Road Traffic Act (1930) the hospital as a voluntary institution, should adopt and charge a flat rate of 8/6d. per day for each person admitted as a result of a car accident.[7]

Appropriate cases of malignant disease were still being treated with radium which was under the care of the lady superintendent who held the key of the radium safe and released the radium to the sister in charge of the ward in which it was to be used.[8] A decade later in 1942 thought was being given to the organisation of cancer treatment on an area basis. Mr David Band on behalf of the honorary medical staff approached the board with the suggestion that all patients requiring radiotherapy be seen in consultation with the surgeon in charge by Dr Robert McWhirter at a central clinic at Edinburgh Royal Infirmary. To facilitate this Dr McWhirter (later Professor McWhirter of the Chair of Medical Radiology of the University of Edinburgh) was appointed consulting radiologist/radiotherapist at Leith Hospital.[9] Obviously it was beginning to be recognised that all hospitals could not offer all therapeutic facilities to all of their patients and in 1938 it was the Medical Chirurgical Society of Edinburgh which proposed to the local authority and the voluntary hospitals in the city the setting up of a committee of enquiry towards the better coordination of hospital services in the Edinburgh area, a concept with which the managers of Leith Hospital were in full agreement.[10]

In 1935 a further, but abortive, attempt to increase the specialist services at the hospital was made. A proposal was put forward that Dr Ninian Bruce, neurologist, and Dr Harrows, psychiatrist establish a "nerve clinic" which would certainly have added to the range of services offered by the hospital but the Board decided to let the matter "lie over".[11] It appears that lack of support from the physicians killed this project.[12]

Even in those days outside bodies or the general public were very willing to raise funds or donate pieces of equipment for medical purposes that had a topical and dramatic appeal. Paralytic poliomyelitis — infantile paralysis — was such a condition at that time and in 1938 the boxing stadium in Mill Lane next to the hospital offered an "iron lung". Dr T. R. R. Todd, senior physician, did not however consider this to be an essential part of the equipment of the hospital and the offer was rejected.[13] Nevertheless when Viscount Nuffield presented this apparatus — a Radcliffe respirator — to the hospital the following year it was gratefully accepted.[14]

Even in 1938 problems with insured and uninsured patients arose necessitating a set of rules to be applied to outpatients. These required that patients be asked if they were insured and if so they had to have a written request from their panel doctor to be examined by the hospital doctor. If it was necessary to prescribe for an insured person medicine was not to be dispensed in the hospital but the prescription taken to the panel doctor for agreement and counter signature before presentation in the usual way to a dispensing chemist. These rules did not apply to accidents or emergencies.[15]

Finance

Taking once again the year 1936, the president, Mr David Bell chairing the annual meeting of the subscribers described the treasurer's financial statement as "very satisfactory".[16] The abstract of accounts (Table 7) gives details of the financial position and some interesting information about where funds came from and how monies were spent. In the hospital annual reports subscriptions and donations were recorded down to 2/6d. (old half crowns) and occupied eleven pages of the report. Contributions from schools, offices, factories, ships and church congregations occupied four pages. The hospital collector visited every household in Leith and in thirty-six pages of double columns the names and addresses of the persons contributing down to single shillings(five new pence) is meticulously set out. In addition to hard cash there were also the pages of gifts of all kinds from eggs to magazines.

Although the deficit of ordinary expenditure over ordinary income for the year 1936 was £2,373 it was, as has been said a generally satisfactory financial position especially as a further appeal for building funds (referred to later) had been launched. Support for charities continued as enthusiastically as ever. 1932 saw Leith Hospital as well as Edinburgh Royal Infirmary sharing the proceeds of Edinburgh student's "rag day" and proceeds from the bridge party and the ball organised by a ladies' committee (and a feature of the local social scene for many years) were again welcomed.[17] The hospital fund committee in the same year raised £3,000 which was used to endow a bed.[18] Three years later however this committee was disbanded and a full time organiser with a committee to assist him was appointed.[19]

Development and Building

Following the success of building the children's wing in the 1920s, thought was given in the early 1930s to the development of ground bought recently in King Street adjacent to ground already owned by the hospital. At the annual meeting of subscribers in 1934 the honorary secretary, Mr R. Beveridge Smith, voiced the opinion that some parts of the hospital particularly the medical wards "were thoroughly out of date" — a view entirely endorsed by the medical staff.[20] He reminded his listeners of the efforts made at the time of Queen Victoria's Diamond Jubilee and suggested that the imminence of another jubilee — the silver jubilee of King George Vth's accession to the throne — would be an appropriate point to launch a further appeal. The following year (1935) a committee had been formed, plans initiated and an appeal launched for £60,000. The objectives of this exercise were quite clear; in addition to the rebuilding of the medical wards additional nurses and maid accommodation and a new eye clinic were proposed.[21] From the start also there was a desire to have paying or private wards, this receiving the full backing of the honorary medical staff and also the unanimous support of general practitioners through the Leith Medical Practitioners Association.[22] The appeal prospered; £8,000 came from Lord Nuffield to endow a ward to be known as the Nuffield ward[23] and a similar sum for a similar purpose from the family of Mr Kenneth Crawford.[24] A radio broadcast appeal on the B.B.C. was made on behalf of the hospital by Lord Salvesen.[25] By 1936 the funds stood at £48,777, by 1937 £61,987 and by 1938 £64,728 when over £18,000 had already been expended on building works. Building was disappointingly delayed however because of repeated alterations to the plans and a considerable rise in building costs and it became clear that a further £40,000 would be needed to complete the whole project.[26] It was decided to proceed initially with the nurses home amidst continuing optimism with regard to financial support and a report in the *Scotsman* of 30th November 1938 promised that the first section would be completed by September 1939. It went on to describe the rooms, each nurse and maid having one of her own, with lounges, dining room and lecture theatre. A "sunshine balcony" was to be built extending between the children's wing and surgical block and the flat roof of the new medical block was to be laid out as a garden. The architect was J. S. Johnston, and appointed as architectural consultant was Mr Tait who, readers were reminded, was responsible for the Empire Exhibition in Glasgow and the recently created Scottish Office buildings on Calton Hill. Regrettably the nurses home was not completed until 1941 and by that time war had put a stop to further building. Post-war conditions and the advent of the National Health Service saw the final demise of the medical ward project but an artist's impression of the building that was being designed, published in the *Edinburgh Evening News* of 20th December 1935 shows what might have been at Leith Hospital [plate 15].

Reference has already been made to Mrs Currie's provision of a convalescent home at Corstorphine. She died in 1919 bequeathing the home to the hospital but in 1935 Miss Campbell M. Currie purchased a house adjoining the original home and gifted it to the hospital. A covered passageway was constructed between the two buildings and the result was a great improvement in convalescent facilities for male and female patients from Leith Hospital.[27] In the same year Mrs James Currie of Larkfield offered to buy, equip and run a house as a convalescent home for children from Leith Hospital at North Berwick.[28] This generous offer was gratefully accepted and as has been mentioned eighty-two children convalesced there in the following year.

Shortly before the onset of war King Street, running between Mill Lane and Great Junction Street, to the east of the main hospital complex was closed to the public so that free access could be had between the ward blocks and nurses home, laundry and kitchens without resorting so much to the subway. This area eventually became an important car park for the hospital.[29]

Staffing of the Hospital

In the pre-war period three physicians, Dr T. R. R. Todd, Dr G. L. Malcolm Smith and Dr D. N. Nicholson were appointed and two surgeons, Mr A. P. Mitchell and Mr R. Leslie Stewart.

Thomas Robert Rushton Todd (1896-1975). He was educated at the Edinburgh Institution when it was at 8 Queen Street now part of the Royal College of Physicians of Edinburgh. His medical studies were interrupted by the first world war when he served with the Scottish Horse Brigade Field Ambulance manned almost entirely by medical students, before being commissioned in the 8th battalion Seaforth Highlanders in France. He graduated M.B. at Edinburgh in 1919, MD ion 1925 and became a Fellow of the Royal College of Physicians of Edinburgh in 1927. For a time he was medical officer to the Rio Tinto mines in Spain before becoming physician to Leith Hospital from 1931 to 1947 and to Queensberry House. Later he became physician to Edinburgh Royal Infirmary retiring in 1961. He was appointed consulting physician to Leith Hospital in 1947.[30]

George Lewis Macolm-Smith (1894-1975), graduated MB at Edinburgh in 1917 and served in the RAMC in the East African campaign being mentioned in dispatches. He became an FRCPE in 1925. After serving as clinical tutor in Edinburgh Royal Infirmary he became assistant physician at Longmore Hospital and physician at Leith Hospital. Retiring in 1959 he continued to work in general practice until two weeks before his death. Before the second world war, as medical officer to the 7th/9th Royal Scots he was asked to set up and command a Scottish field hospital. He went to France in 1939 and although left behind at the Dunkirk evacuation managed to return to the United Kingdom shortly afterwards.[31]

Douglas Nairn Nicholson (1902-1976). Graduating in 1926 he became FRCPE in 1931. He became assistant physician at Leith Hospital and physician for diseases of children at the New Town Dispensary. He decided to specialise in paediatrics and became a lecturer in the subject at Edinburgh University. In addition to his appointment as physician at Leith Hospital he held appointments as consultant physician at the Royal Hospital for Sick Children Edinburgh and the Princess Margaret Rose Hospital. In the second world war he commanded the medical division of a military hospital and was mentioned in dispatches. He was a member of the Royal Company of Archers, the Sovereign's bodyguard in Scotland.[32]

Alexander Philp Mitchell (1885-1959). He had a distinguished under-graduate career being awarded the McCunn scholarship in surgery and graduating MB at Edinburgh in 1907. He proceeded to the MD in 1909, FRCSE in 1912 and was awarded the gold medal for his ChM thesis in 1913. For five years he acted as private assistant to Sir Harold Stiles and as a captain in the RAMC in the first world war, served at Bangour and Craigleith Hospitals gaining wide experience in orthopaedic and traumatic surgery. He had expertise in surgical tuberculosis in children. He was successively assistant surgeon at Leith Hospital and surgeon to the children's wing and general surgical unit. Later in his career, he did work at Hartwood Asylum investigating and operating on cases requiring leukotomy.[33]

Robert Leslie Stewart (?-1981). He graduated M.B. at Edinburgh in 1917 and served in the Royal Navy before becoming FRCSE and successively clinical tutor, assistant surgeon and surgeon to Edinburgh Royal Infirmary. As well as surgeon to Leith Hospital, he was honorary urological consultant at Dunfermline and West Fife Hospital and consultant surgeon to the Royal Navy in Scotland.[34]

Assistant physicians included Dr J. A. Bruce — later to be appointed physician, Dr R. M. Murray Lyon and Dr H. L. Wallace who became the first professor of paediatrics in the university of Natal. Assistant surgeons were Mr David Band and Mr J. R. Cameron, both later becoming surgeons, and Mr John Bruce.

The gynaecologist appointed at this time was E. C. Fahmy.

Ernest Chalmers Fahmy (1892-1982). Born in China he graduated MB at Edinburgh University in 1918 his studies having been interrupted by service in the Royal Artillery in the first world war when he was wounded. After post graduate study in Vienna he became FRCSE in 1925 and later FRCPE and FRCOG. In addition to being gynaecologist to Leith Hospital he was obstetrician and gynaecologist to

Edinburgh Royal Infirmary. He was a contributor to Baird's *"Combined Textbook of Obstetrics and Gynaecology"*. He was appointed consulting gynaecologist to Leith Hospital in 1947.[35]

G. I. Scott,later to be appointed to the chair of ophthalmology at Edinburgh University, was appointed ophthalmic surgeon. C. E. Scott was appointed ENT surgeon. Miss D. A. D. Bannerman became anaesthetist in 1931 and Dr J. B. King and Dr J. J. Kinnimonth were appointed radiologists in 1931 and 1937 respectively.

Charles Ernest Scott (1895-1957). His medical studies at Edinburgh were interrupted by service in the Royal Navy in the first world war and he graduated MB in 1921. He took his FRCSE in 1926 and became assistant and clinical tutor to Dr J. Lithgow's unit in Edinburgh Royal Infirmary. Later he was assistant to Dr Douglas Guthrie at the Royal Hospital for Sick Children, Edinburgh and then surgeon to Leith Hospital and surgeon with responsibility for ENT services in the Borders. He was a keen rugby player in his youth and curler in his later years.[36]

A consulting dental surgeon, D. L. G. Radford was appointed in 1931. Three pathologists, Bruce M. Dick, John Bruce and R. F. Ogilvie were appointed in this time, the first two being in fact surgeons and later to achieve eminence in that field. In reality the duties apportioned to the assistants were slightly complicated. For example, Mr John Bruce as assistant surgeon also undertook the surgical pathology and supervised the massage department; Mr J. R. Cameron as assistant surgeon also performed the duties of registrar and one of the assistant physicians undertook the medical pathology.[37] The assistant surgeon in the ENT department was Mr A. B. Smith and in the gynaecology department were Dr J. Bruce Dewar and Edwin Robertson who left in 1939 to occupy the chair of obstetrics and gynaecology at Queens University, Kingston, Ontario.[38]

Although it was as far back as 1912 that the honorary medical staff drew the attention of the managers to the advisability of having a skin specialist appointed[39] it was not until 1931 when the first dermatologist was appointed. Dr Robert Aitken served from 1931 to 1936 when he was succeeded by Dr Grant Peterkin.

Robert Aitken (1888-1954). Graduating in 1911 he was highly commended for his MD thesis awarded in 1915. He became FRCPE in 1921. He first worked as a general practitioner before specialising in dermatology and became physician to Leith Hospital, Edinburgh Royal Infirmary and Perth Infirmary. He published two books one on *"Ultraviolet Radiations and Their Uses"* and *"The Problems of Lupus Vulgaris"*. The Royal Society of Edinburgh elected him a fellow in 1945.[40]

George Alexander Grant Peterkin (1906-1987). Following his graduation as MB ChB at Edinburgh in 1929 he studied dermatology at Copenhagen and became a specialist in skin diseases at Edinburgh Royal Infirmary, Leith Hospital, Deaconess Hospital and Bangour

Hospital. He joined the RAMC in 1942 as a dermatologist and served with the First Army in Algeria and Naples where he was in charge of 1,000 beds for skin diseases. He was awarded the MBE and by the Americans the medal of freedom with bronze palms. In 1937 he was the first to report infection of human skin with orf virus and was co-editor with R. Cranstone Lowe of the textbook *"Common Diseases of the Skin"*. He was a keen antiquarian and wrote a book on Scottish dovecots.[41]

It was in 1934 that thought was first given to altering the day to day administration and control of the hospital by the appointment of a medical superintendent (the minutes of the Board of Managers specified a "male medical superintendent"). Miss Wise, the lady super-intendent, was to retire in 1935 and in July 1934 Sister Inglis, it was decided, should be appointed "matron" on Miss Wise's departure to run the hospital until a medical superintendent was appointed.[43] In March the following year, for reasons that are not clear, the decision to appoint a medical superintendent was rescinded and Miss Inglis was appointed lady superintendent at a salary of £250 per annum.[44] Another eight years were to pass before this matter was raised again.

No important changes had occurred in the work of residents or nurses in this time. Fifth year medical students were appointed as clinical assistants to the residents[45] and the residents' posts continued to be very popular. This was mainly because of the abundance of work of all kinds but perhaps the generosity of a local brewer by which each resident was allotted a bottle of beer per day had some bearing also. Residents from other not so liberal hospitals would sometimes assist the Leith residents with the task of disposing of these at weekends![46] The nurses were governed by a set of rules some of which seem restrictive by modern standards and are reproduced below.

Rules for Nurses

1. No nurse is to be in any ward except in the performance of her duty, or to have there an attaché-case. No nurse is to leave a ward during her hours of duty there without the permission of the ward sister.
2. Each nurse must be punctual according to her timetable.
3. No nurse is to be absent from a meal without having given notice of her intention not to be present to the home sister.
4. After 10.30 p.m. no day nurse, and after 12.30 p.m. no night nurse, is to be in the bedroom of another nurse.
5. Lights in all nurses' bedrooms must be extinguished not later than 11.15 p.m.
6. Each nurse must keep her bedroom tidy and be responsible for the safety of her own property, in the event of the loss of which the hospital will not indemnify her.

7. No article belonging to the hospital is to be removed by a nurse from the dining room, sitting rooms or classroom, unless permission to remove it is granted by the home sister.

8. Any nurse who is not feeling well is to report her condition to the home sister.

9. No nurse is to consult any doctor either attached or not attached to the hospital without the permission of the lady superintendent.

10. Talking is forbidden on the stairs or corridors of the hospital.

11. No nurse is to accept a personal gift from a patient.

12. Smoking is forbidden in the hospital. In the nurses' home it is permitting only in the sitting room.

13. No nails or pins are to be driven into the walls of bedrooms. No light other than electric is to be used there and no fire is to be lighted.

14. Nurses are forbidden to turn on the water in a bath and then to leave it unattended.

15. Nurses are to arrange to have all their correspondence addressed to the Nurses' home.

16. Nurses are not to receive visitors during their hours of duty, nor are they to show them through the wards without permission from the lady superintendent.

17. "Long leave" and "early leave" passes are granted by the lady superintendent between 9 a.m. and 10 a.m. Nurses who are late in coming in shall report themselves to the night sister when they return.

18. Nurses are to exercise the strictist economy in the use of all hospital stores, and to take the greatest care of all hospital equipment.

It may be added that a new set of rules for the resident medical officers was made about the same time. They are not remarkable for the times although one wonders what circumstances necessitated rule 23 which stated: "The relations between the residents and the nurses shall be strictly official!" Present day house officers might also raise an eyebrow at rule 2 which states: "No salary shall be attached to any of the offices except such honorarium as the managers may from time to time decide" and rule 4: "No resident shall be entitled to leave of absence (except on account of illness duly certified), but should he obtain a further appointment he shall before entering upon it be entitled to a holiday of fourteen days."

Although Leith Hospital was by this time a recognised teaching school for nurses, no prizes were available before 1936. Mrs Langwill, an Edinburgh Royal Infirmary trained nurse and wife of Dr Langwill, a consulting physician to the hospital, was amazed to learn of this deficiency and that year donated money for prizes. It was the wish of the nurses themselves that medals be given and Dr Langwill (Mrs Langwill being ill) presented the first silver medal to nurse Isabella Beattie and bronze medals (second equal) to nurses Jean Todd and Joan McLeod.[47]

In 1933 a proposal was made that a lady almoner be appointed but a decision was not taken following a letter to the managers from Mrs Currie, president of the Samaritan Society, a matter which will be referred to later. The following year a part-time radiographer was appointed at a wage of £5 per week.[48]

Royal Occasions and Trade Union Concerns

Leith Hospital like other institutions in the Edinburgh area was accustomed to visits from the Sovereign's annual representative, the Lord High Commissioner, to the General Assembly of the Church of Scotland. It had never had a royal visit however and the visit of the Duke and Duchess of Kent in 1935 caused great excitement in the town and gave much satisfaction to the hospital. The president, Mr David Bell, hoped that it would not be long before another royal visit was made obviously referring to the opening of the proposed new hospital building and extension.[50] The *Edinburgh and Leith Observer* of 31st May of that year describes the enthusiastic reception given to the Duke and Duchess who visited male and female surgical wards and the children's wards. A photograph [plate 16] records the visit to the children's wing; the name of the child is unknown — could it have been Charlie Cormack whose broken clockwork engine the Duke according to the newspaper attempted to repair?

Two years later the hospital was visited by the Duchess of Gloucester. It had been a busy and crowded visit for her and the Duke. He had laid the foundation stone of the government offices on Calton Hill, she had received the freedom of the city of Edinburgh in the morning and visited Leith Hospital and presided at a meeting of the Queen's Institute of District Nursing in the afternoon.[51]

1937 was also the year of the coronation of King George VI and Queen Elizabeth. To mark this Mr and Mrs Gilbert Archer (he was by then president of the board of managers) presented coronation china mugs to all the children in the hospital[52] and also erected a stand in Taylor Gardens so that the managers, medical and nursing staff, patients and others could view the royal motor drive through Leith.[53]

In contrast to the pleasure of royal occasions displeasure was being expressed by trades union bodies about this time. At the annual meeting of subscribers in 1933, Councillor Cathcart raised the issue of representation on the board of management of the Edinburgh District Trades and Labour Council; he was advised that this should be discussed at the next meeting of the board of managers.[54] Clearly no action was taken as in 1935 a letter was received from this body again raising the issue, the answer being that nominations could be made at the meeting of subscribers.[55] It will be remembered that the board of managers had representation from the town council, Leith dock commission, honorary medical officers and clergy; in 1938 it was pointed out by the chairman when two remaining vacancies were being filled at the subscribers meeting that for many years there had been a very happy arrangement with the local shipyard workers whereby they put forward the name of a representative for the consideration of the board each term. Mr Minor had been such a member of the board for some years.[56] Such an arrangement was not to the liking of the trades council and it returned to the attack in 1939 demanding the right to have their representative on the board. The demand was resisted however and with the onset of war this affair was submerged under other pressing matters.

War — Once Again

General Problems

In their report to the managers for 1938 the honorary medical staff recorded their appreciation of the arrangements made for dealing with events that might arise out of possible air raids. Air raid precautions that year were pursued by the installation of pumps on the recommendations of the fire brigade and bags and material for covering windows were purchased.[58] As war became imminent in 1939 the theatre windows were darkened and other preparations hastened but three weeks after the declaration of war ARP work was not yet completed although "every effort was being made".[59]

The hospital had to cope with a number of unusual demands and circumstances. Routine work was immediately affected by the Department of Health's instruction that the hospital be cleared of all inpatients on 30th August 1939 except those too ill to be moved.[60] For many weeks admissions were limited to emergencies only. Under the appropriate emergency regulations the managers had been instructed to reserve 107 beds for the use of civilian cases and 100 beds for civilian and service casualties[61] (which of course did not materialise as anticipated), the increase in the bed complement of the hospital being achieved by adding ten beds to each ward. Dr A. M. Wood, one of the hospital's retired consulting physicians, accepted the invitation to coordinate the air raid casualty services at the hospital.[62] The hospital was also required to construct an emergency theatre and sterilising room which caused some controversy as the instruments which had been requested from the Department of Health were not supplied. They were not necessary said the department as the hospital was intended only as a casualty clearing hospital, an explanation which the managers found far from satisfactory.[63] Equipment had to be bought for a rescue and repair section established at the hospital[64] and a gas decontamination centre constructed at the front entrance to the hospital.[65] The staffing of this centre was in the charge of Dr R. F. Ogilvie with a team of hospital nurses and auxiliary nurses.[66] There was a loss of amenity when the convalescent home for children at North Berwick was requisitioned by the military authorities and part of the convalescent house at Corstorphine was used as an air raid warden's post.[67] But the ubiquitous air raid shelter was, in the hospital, painted and by 1943 used as part of the massage department!

In addition to coping with these problems staff had, in the early part of the war, to carry gas masks[68] and to provide fire watchers under a Fire Prevention Order. A minimum of fifteen fire watchers had to be provided for the hospital and they of course required beds and bedding and were paid at a rate of 3/- per night.[69] Such measures were not superfluous as Leith received more attention from German bombers in the second world war than it had from Zeppelins in the first. In March and April 1941 raids on towns in east and south east Scotland with high explosive and incendiary bombs caused considerable blast and fire damage to many including Leith. This time the hospital did not escape although damage was not severe.[70] Financially this was covered by war damage insurance[71] and later in 1943 there are records of several hundreds of pounds being received in compensation from the War Damage Commission.[72]

One incident which cheered the entire British population in the uncertain days of 1940, which affected the hospital, was the *"Altmark"* affair. This German vessel carrying British prisoners, mainly from merchant vessels sunk in the south Atlantic, to Germany was intercepted and boarded in Norwegian waters by the destroyer *H.M.S. Cossack.* The prisoners were landed at Leith, the hospital attending to medical problems, which prompted an anonymous donor to give a substantial sum towards the rebuilding of the medical wards and the dedication of a bed "To commemorate the exploit of the rescue of the prisoners on the Altmark by the ship's company of H.M.S. Cossack".[73]

Effects on the Work of the Hospital

One of the early effects on hospital work was the large increase in the numbers of outpatients seen in 1940 in contrast to 1939. The reasons identified by medical staff for this were firstly the increase in employment, secondly the increase in overtime worked with thereby the potential for stress and injury and lastly the fact that patients were being discharged earlier and asked to attend the outpatient department.[74] The inpatient load also increased and of course included service patients which was not without its problems. They caused difficulties it was alleged by being of a more lively disposition and wanting to smoke, talk and walk about when it was inconvenient for others![75] Again precise numbers of service patients treated are unavailable although particular reference is made to the wounded admitted after D Day.[76] By that time disquiet was being expressed about the exclusion of civilian patients urgently in need of treatment and it was suggested that service patients be admitted only as emergencies. This, it was pointed out, might be counter productive as the Department of Health might withdraw some trained nurses of which Leith Hospital was allowed more than otherwise to cope with the service men.[77] Merchant seamen of many nationalities were also treated particular mention being made by Mr Norman Salvesen, the Norwegian consul, of the Norwegian government's appreciation of the numbers of Norwegian seamen attended to.[78]

By 1943 there was a considerable waiting list for non-urgent operations. For example 235 persons were waiting for ENT operations and an attempt was made to provide additional beds and also to enlist the help of EMS hospitals. But as Dr Scott, the ENT surgeon pointed out, he would have had to operate on them there instead of at Leith Hospital.[79] Just after the war, in 1947 reference was made to the decrease in ENT operations carried out due to the epidemic of poliomyelitis in progress at that time.[80] Reference has been made to the increase in outpatient numbers and the causes of this. The pressure of heavy work in shipyards, docks and factories resulted in a large number of hand injuries, a particularly serious factor in curtailing available manpower during a total war effort. For this reason the hospital established a special hand clinic.[81] One of the temporary assistant surgeons, Mr A. R. Murray, was in charge of this and with the essential co-operation of the physiotherapy department which in 1943 became officially known as such rather than the massage department, impressive results were obtained.

With the numbers of service men and sailors in a busy port in war time it was perhaps inevitable that the matter of treatment of venereal diseases would again be raised. This time pressure came from the Port Welfare Committee and the Leith Ship Owner's Society to establish a clinic at the hospital. Medical staff and managers after discussion with the medical officer for health and identification of accommodation and staff required decided that it would be impossible as well as undesirable to start such a clinic at Leith Hospital and suggested that it be established at Seafield Hospital (the Eastern General Hospital).[82]

Medical and Nursing Difficulties

At the beginning of the war the honorary medical staff requested an end to the practice of pathology being carried out by either medical or surgical clinicians. As mentioned before Dr Robertson Ogilvie was appointed in 1939 with an honorarium of £25 per annum.[83] Later he was to have the assistance of Dr Blackwood and Dr Campbell for the duration of the war.[84]

Many members of all staff left for war service. By early 1940 the hospital was understaffed medically and surgically[85] and the assistance of third, fourth and fifth year medical students was welcomed, the lady

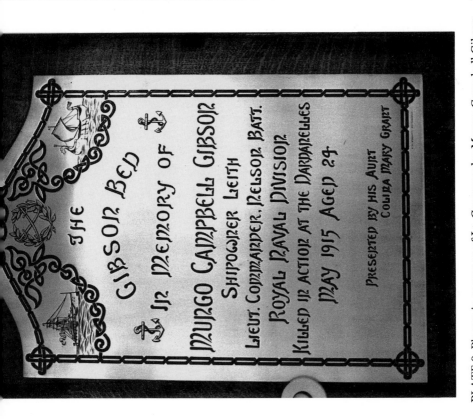

THE GIBSON BED

In Memory of

MUNGO CAMPBELL GIBSON
SHIPOWNER LEITH
LIEUT. COMMANDER, NELSON BATT.
ROYAL NAVAL DIVISION
KILLED IN ACTION AT THE DARDANELLES
MAY 1915 AGED 29

PRESENTED BY HIS AUNT
LOUISA MARY GRANT

To the Glory of God

and

For the Relief of Human Suffering

THIS BED has been ENDOWED

by

Public Subscription

In Memory of:

The Gallant Officers
Non-Commissioned Officers and Men
of the
Leith Territorial Regiment
The 7th Batt. Royal Scots

who perished on
22nd May 1915
in a
Railway Accident
at
Gretna
on their way to
Gallipoli

PLATE 9. Plaque in memory of Lt. Commander Mungo Campbell Gibson   PLATE 10. Plaque in memory of those killed in the Gretna rail disaster

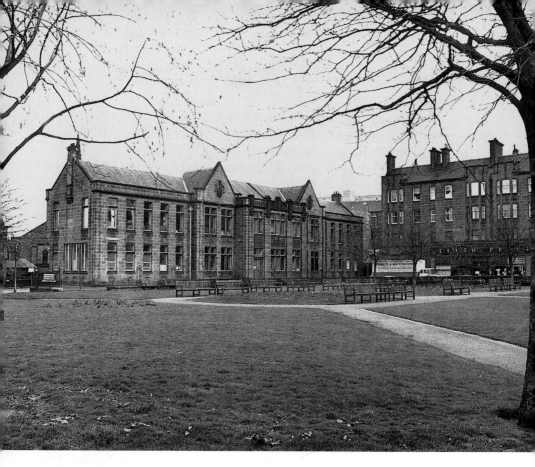

PLATE 11. Leith Hospital. Children's Wing. Leith's 1914-18 War Memorial, seen from Taylor Gardens

PLATE 12. Sketch plan of Leith Hospital site in the 1920s and 30s

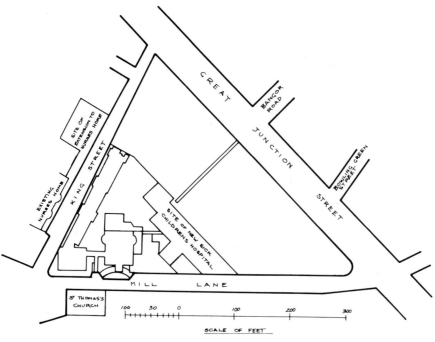

BLOCK PLAN OF SITE

superintendent supplying them with meals.[86] Two years later the managers were seriously concerned about the efficiency of the hospital as the
number of qualified residents had been reduced to two[87] and the same
year they had the sad task of recording the death on active service of
Dr Ronald Stewart, one of the residents who had just finished his duties
at Leith Hospital.[88] During the course of the war temporary assistants
were appointed amongst whom were Mr J. F. Curr and Mr A. R.
Murray in surgery, Dr Ethna W. Little in gynaecology, Dr H. K. Dastur
in ENT surgery and Dr C. R. D. Leeds in ophthalmology. In 1941 a Mr
Lumsden was appointed dental officer, Dr Radford's services being
retained for maxillo-facial surgery[89] and in the same year a resident surgical officer (RSO) Mr Tulloch, was appointed.[90] The most significant
appointment, however, was that of Dr Norman Carmichael in 1943 as
the first medical superintendent of Leith Hospital.[91] It had been
decided initially that on the retirement of Miss Inglis, the lady superintendent, a temporary replacement would be made and then a part-time
medical superintendent appointed who would be assisted by a matron
responsible for nursing and nursing training only. The office bearers
were convinced that a medical superintendent was necessary to exercise
proper control over resident medical and surgical staff and the appointment was made by November of that year with Miss A. M. McKee as
"matron and deputy superintendent". Perhaps the managers were
influenced by what they saw as a "breach of discipline" by the resident
doctors in 1940, the matter earning their slightly censorious disap-
proval being the attachment to the top of the hospital flag pole of a pair
of pyjamas![92]

The task that Miss McKee accepted must have been a particularly
difficult one in the light of staff and material shortages and the peculiar
difficulties of war time. There was some support for nursing staff from
the civil nursing reserve[93] and in 1941 the age of probationer nurses
starting training was reduced from nineteen to eighteen years.[94] Some
women were accepted for training at Leith Hospital as the result of a
letter from the Co-ordinating Committee for Refugees in 1939 which
asked that war refugees from Europe be given opportunities to qualify
as nurses.[95] Assistance with nursing training was also given to Liberton
Hospital[96] and Longmore Hospital[97] by a system of affiliation which
allowed a total of eight probationers being accepted per year.

It is very much to the credit of the managers that in the midst of war
they presented a memorandum which embodied an imaginative and
progressive idea with regard to nurses. They resolved to open a preliminary training course for girls of sixteen and a half to bridge the gap
between leaving school and starting nursing training.[95] Theoretical and
practical subjects would be taught by a sister tutor, at evening classes if
need be and in addition instruction by hospital staff in laundry work,
cooking, kitchen work and housekeeping would be given. They were to
be allocated a room in the nurses home and board from Monday to

Friday. Details of the scheme were submitted to the Scottish Education Department and the General Nursing Council for approval. The annual report for 1945 however had to record that this was still mainly an idea and deplored the short-sighted policy of failure to provide an adequate number of sister tutors.

The Approach to the National Health Service

At the end of the war in 1945 only three more years were left to Leith as a voluntary hospital. It had been realised for many years that a scheme of co-ordination of hospitals in cities was required; indeed it was the honorary medical staff of the hospital who in 1936 said that such was required in Edinburgh "on grounds of efficiency and economy".[99] In 1941 the annual meeting of the court of contributors was addressed by the Countess of Rosbery (who was closely associated with a hospital of similar size in the south of England) in which she warned of the financial climate which would affect voluntary hospitals in the future. "I should hate to be thought a wet blanket" she said "but I take a very gloomy view of the financial future of voluntary hospitals. Unless all are prepared to join some scheme of inter-dependence of this sort [the Nuffield Provincial Hospitals Trust] surely their days are numbered." The following year the managers in their report alluding to the Beveridge report and referring to the assumption in it of a complete medical service said, "Nothing could be more desirable and in our view it would be wrong for us as a body concerned with the health of the people of Leith not to say so". There was therefore an atmosphere of realism albeit reluctant and sad. This was underlined by the treasurer's remarks in 1946 when he stated, "It must be evident to the Board from an examination of the treasurer's abstracts of accounts over the past few years that without substantial government grants the hospital in a very short time cannot carry on."[100]

Activities in the Last Years of the Voluntary Hospital

Despite the uncertainty clinical work increased as can be seen from the 1946 statistics (Table 6). Curiously there was a considerable decrease that year in attendances at surgical outpatient department compared with the previous two or three years. Reasons identified by the surgical staff were: 1. Fracture cases were now being seen at a special clinic. 2. Penicillin had reduced the number of treatments required. 3. A fall in the length of working hours and the number of accidents. 4. The honorary staff were insisting on patients bringing a doctor's letter. 5. The hand clinic had ceased and, 6. It was the modern practice to dress wounds less frequently.[101] The following year a drop in attendance at the ENT clinic was reported, a circumstance attributed to the use of penicillin.[102] It is difficult for modern clinicians to appreciate the importance and impact of penicillin at that time. One member of staff (Mr Murray in 1945) was appointed officer in charge of penicillin and there was some anxiety when in 1946 the Department of Health announced that the free supply of penicillin would cease at the end of May. The managers calculated that at the present rate of consumption it would cost £120 per month to supply this antibiotic and it urged medical staff to restrict its use.[103] Another department which increased its workload at this time was the physiotherapy department due mainly to an increase in the treatment of fractures and a special clinic for this purpose.[104]

During the war in 1943 an electrocardiograph was purchased secondhand from Edinburgh Royal Infirmary for £150.[105] Four years later it was reported to be defective and should only be used by a skilled person. The solution was not to replace it but to get one of the ECG technicians at the Edinburgh Royal Infirmary to instruct Miss Auchmuty in its use![106]

It had been agreed that the hospital should not establish its own laboratory, but by 1946 the Royal College of Physicians of Edinburgh laboratory was complaining that the hospital's contribution was insufficient and the medical superintendent was instructed to negotiate an appropriate sum. By that time also the hospital was making a contribution to the pathology department of the University of Edinburgh for pathological and histological work carried out in its laboratory.[107]

In 1940 numbers 4 and 5 Mill Lane were bought by the hospital.[108] This property, on the opposite side of the lane to the hospital, consisted of a house, a small confectionary factory and ground and it was proposed to use it for a residency for doctors and a completely new building for the physiotherapy department.[109] When tenders were invited in 1947 for appropriate alterations they were deemed to be disappointingly high[110] and the following year the Department of Health for Scotland withdrew its support for the project with the result that the managers were unable to obtain a licence for the work to be carried out. This had a "knock-on" effect as the opening of new wards was dependent on accommodation for additional nurses being available in rooms vacated by resident medical staff.[111] Eventually these premises were converted for the use of all outpatient clinics at the hospital, secretaries rooms and a records department.

After the war the hospital lost its convalescent facilities. The children's convalescent home at North Berwick was sold as it was decided that the hospital could not run it with proper supervision[112] and the Corstorphine home was similarly disposed of.

Several members of medical staff were appointed just before the start of the National Health Service; Dr J. A. Bruce as physician, Dr W. A. Liston as gynaecologist, Dr C. R. D. Leeds as ophthalmic surgeon and Mr David Band and Mr J. R. Cameron as surgeons. Drs A. W. Wright and J. B. Buchanan were appointed assistant physicians, Messrs A. F. M. Barron, J. A. Ross, T. I. Wilson and D. McIntosh assistant surgeons, Dr A. F. Anderson, assistant gynaecologist, Dr G. S. Dhillon, assistant ophthalmologist and Dr L. L. Theron, assistant anaesthetist.

John Alistair Bruce (1905-1972). Becoming a fellow of the Royal College of Physicians of Edinburgh in 1934 he served the College as treasurer for eleven years and a vice president from 1963-1966. He became physician to Leith Hospital just before the advent of the National Health Service and then physician to the Eastern General Hospital and Roodlands Hospital. He was principal medical officer to the Scottish Life Assurance Company. A keen territorial army officer in the 78 Field Regiment Royal Artillery before the war he was compulsorily transferred to the RAMC and served in Egypt and Iraq. His father and grandfather before him had been high constables of Holyrood House and so was he, serving as moderator in 1969.[113]

David Band (1901-1988). He qualified in 1923 and became an FRCSE in 1926. In 1935 he was appointed lecturer in clinical surgery in the University of Edinburgh and later became reader in urology. He was an internationally renowned urological surgeon particularly for his work on urogenital tuberculosis. He was elected an FRSE in 1950, and served as a councillor of the RCSE for thirteen years.[114]

William Alexander Liston (1909-1962). Having graduated MB at Edinburgh in 1933 he was on the staff of Edinburgh Royal Infirmary before the war when he was an active officer in a territorial army unit. On the outbreak of war he insisted on remaining with a combatant unit and served with the Royal Artillery in Burma being awarded the Military Cross. It was not until 1945 that he transferred to the RAMC. In 1946 he resumed appointment at Edinburgh Royal Infirmary and also had appointments at Leith Hospital, Bangour Hospital and later the Eastern General Hospital. As well as being a Fellow of the Royal College of Obstetricians and Gynaecologists he was elected a Fellow of the Royal College of Physicians of Edinburgh in 1947.[115]

Charles Rupert Duncan Leeds (1905-1966). After graduating MB at Edinburgh in 1928 he entered general practice at Gretna. While there he decided to specialise in ophthalmology and took his DOMS and FRCSE in 1937. He was assistant to the Royal London Ophthalmic Hospital and then to the Edinburgh Royal Infirmary. As well as surgeon to Leith Hospital he was surgeon to Dunfermline and West Fife Hospital. He was interested in sport and music being a keen rugby player and golfer and he played both the organ and piano.[116]

In 1946 the medical staff approved in principle the appointment of paediatric physicians and paediatric surgeons but Dr D. N. Nicholson continued to undertake the medical duties and for a brief period in 1945 and 1946 the paediatric surgeon was Mr John Bruce (later Sir John and professor of surgery at Edinburgh University).[117] In the same year the honorary medical staff agreed to the appointment of up to six supernumerary class 1 (house officer) and class 2 (registrar) medical officers at Leith Hospital.[118] These posts were provided for demobilised service medical officers returning to civilian practice.

1947 also saw a new departure with regard to the honorary medical staff which was the granting by the managers of honoraria to the senior doctors who felt that honorary work was no longer necessary. The sum of £250 per annum was agreed.[119]

It is perhaps sad that the last years of the voluntary hospital witnessed disagreement between the managers and local clergy. A letter from the Leith Ministers Fraternal in 1946 requested the appointment of a hospital chaplain who would receive an honorarium. The managers however thought that the appointment of a protestant minister to a hospital which served such a large Roman Catholic population was undesirable[120] but when the ministers produced facts and figures (only 10-12 per cent of inpatients in Leith Hospital being Roman Catholic) the managers reluctantly agreed.[121] Nevertheless a slight degree of discord persisted as in May 1948 the Fraternal was protesting about the restrictions that had been imposed on visiting ministers to 2-4 p.m. daily and exclusion from the children's wards.[122] The matter does not appear to have been resolved before the dissolution of the board of management.

The Advent of the National Health Service

Discussion of the proposal for a National Health Service started of course during the war. A resolution accepted at a conference of voluntary hospitals in 1944 expressed full sympathy with the government's intention to secure a coordinated hospital and consultant service and to make such a service accessible to any member of the community regardless of income but viewed with grave concern the proposals with regard to administration and finance. Leith Hospital managers making comments on the white paper which preceeded the act said that the only acceptable solution appeared to be a direct payment to voluntary hospitals from the exchequer sufficient to meet a reasonable proportion of the necessary expenditure leaving these hospitals as voluntary agencies.[123] This now seems a somewhat unrealistic view.

It is also difficult to assess the purpose of a questionnaire sent by the hospital to the people of Leith. 1400 replies were in favour of nationalisation of the hospital and 5600 against. This information was passed to local members of parliament, the Secretary of State for Scotland and the press.[124]

The ultimate outcome was of course inevitable and the managers saw to it that the handover went smoothly. They aimed as they said in their last report "at presenting to the appropriate authority on the 5th July 1948 a hospital well staffed, well equipped and well deserving of the praise that had been bestowed on it in the past".[125] In his final statement the treasurer recorded the position of the hospital's funds as standing at £198,984 which included endowment and special purposes monies of £176,876. He estimated the value of the hospital buildings, contents and equipment as being not less than £700,000. It was however the handing over of endowments of over £170,000 which had been expressly bequeathed to Leith Hospital for the benefit of the people of Leith that was particularly disturbing to the managers and indeed to the community of Leith.

At the final meeting of the court of contributors of Leith Hospital on the 27th February 1948 the adoption of the report was moved by General Sir Philip Christison (grandson of Sir Robert Christison who had occupied the chair of materia medica at Edinburgh University) but it was seconded by one of the most distinguished of many distinguished former members of the staff of the hospital — Sir Henry Wade. He made a moving speech making reference to his own early involvement of the hospital. "Here in this hospital" he said "the keel of my career was laid and down the slipway it was launched. I wish now after so many years to thank those managers who for better or for worse chose me to be a member of the staff and particularly I want to say how fortunate I was in being associated with so brilliant colleagues. First of all I had then as my senior colleague a Leith born man of great eminence Mr Alexander Miles and I learned from Miles what surgery is." Speaking on the future he said "I say this, that if the individuality, the personality and the attraction of Leith Hospital are seriously damaged it will be a bad thing and a misfortune for the nation."

The curtain can be lowered most appropriately on this long and important century of Leith Hospital's existence by quoting the notice which appeared in the *Scotsman* of 3rd July 1948.

Leith Hospital (Incorporated)
1848 - 1948

This hospital uniting the Leith Fever Hospital, Humane Society, Dispensary and Casualty Hospital in 1848 has for 100 years been maintained by the voluntary subscriptions and service of Leith people.

The managers record this and the thanks due to all those who have co-operated in this great social achievement — voluntary, inspiring and successful — to be ended 5th July 1948.

W. D. T. Green, President.

C. M. S. Whitelaw, Vice-President and Honorary Secretary.

R. L. Gorrie, Honorary Treasurer.

TABLE 6

Inpatient and Outpatient Statistics 1936 and 1946

	1936		1946	
Inpatients	Adult	Paediatric	Adult	Paediatric
Surgical	764	264	1042	370
Medical	421	288	555	375
Gynaecological	273	—	259	—
Ophthalmic	64	22	58	12
Ear, nose and throat	375	254	180	493
	1897	828	2094	1250
Operations				
Surgical	484	170	775	181
Gynaecological	230	—	235	—
Ophthalmic	29	2	44	8
Ear, nose and throat	326	240	158	328
	1069	412	1212	517
Outpatients (new patients)				
Surgical	10,750†		14,862†	
Medical	2972		2246	
Gynaecological	1008		527	
Ophthalmic	1341		986	
Ear, nose and throat	1293		1542	
Dermatological	563*		627	
Physiotherapy	349		517	
Fracture clinic	—		499	
	18,276+		21,806+	
Operations in OPD				
Surgical	475		864	
ENT	64		100	
	539		964	
X-Ray Department				
Number of radiographs	4121		7885	
Number of patients	2788		5623	
Ultra-Violet Radiation				
Total treatments given	10,747		6144	

*   Not a full year.
+   In 1936 a total of 74,788 return patients were seen and in 1946, 78,040.
†   Includes "casualty" attendances.

TABLE 7

ABSTRACT OF TREASURER'S ACCOUNTS
For Year 1936

RECEIPTS

A.   Ordinary Income.

I.   Annual Subscriptions and Donations

Per Treasurer..	£3309 9 8	
Per Treasurer, School, Office etc.	175 15 7	
Per Treasurer, Boxes in Hospital............	829 14 4	
	£4314 19 7	
Per collector...	757 8 7	£5072 8 2

II.   Central Funds

Leith Hospital Flag Day.........................	£1136 14 2	
Edinburgh University Students Represen-tative Council Charities Committee...	200 11 5	£1337 5 7

III. Congregational &c. Collections   £350 19 6

IV. Employees' Collections

Per Treasurer...	£1617 9 9	
Per Collector...	900 1 5	£2517 11 2

V.   Grants from Public Bodies

Edinburgh Corporation.........................	£150 0 0	
Edinburgh Education Authority............	74 0 0	
Leith Industrial School Trustees............	100 0 0	
Leith Dock Commission	300 0 0	£624 0 0

VI.   Invested Property

Dividends, Interest, Feuduties, etc.........	£5635 18 10	
Cottage Home Endowment Interest......	29 13 0	
Income Tax Refund...............................	1478 9 0	£7144 0 10

VII. Receipts on Account of Services to Patients   £203 13 8

VIII. Other Receipts

Cottage Home	£27 5 0	
Stead Benefaction.................................	380 17 11	
Miscellaneous	151 1 0	£559 3 11

                                                   £17,809 2 10

B.   Extraordinary Income.

I.   Free Legacies   £4222 2 1

II.   For Endowment of Beds or Special Purposes   £11,512 5 6

Total Funds at close of 1935

Leith Hospital Ordinary Funds	£17,443 3 10	
Leith Hospital Bed Endowment	75,683 12 0	
Leith Hospital Cot Endowment	3,500 0 0	
Leith Hospital Cottage Home Endowment	847 18 11	
Leith Hospital Outpatient Endowment	1,069 4 11	
Leith Hospital David Ferguson Endowment for Eye Department	38,000 0 0	
Leith Hospital A. Mackie for Children's Wing	100 0 0	
Leith Hospital Miss C. M. Currie's Endowment — Cottage Home	137 0 0	
Leith Hospital Leith Churches Wireless Fund	160 0 0	
Leith War Memorial (Children's Wing)	26,708 19 6	£163,649 19 2

£192,971 7 6

EXPENDITURE

A. MAINTENANCE

I. Provisions

Meat	£852 19 7	
Bread	372 14 3	
Groceries	1203 16 10	
Fish	213 13 3	
Milk	869 8 7	
Vegetables and Fruit	287 7 1	
Cottage Home	265 10 2	
		£4,065 9 9

II. Surgery and Dispensary

Drugs	£1378 3 3	
Dressings	446 10 4	
Instruments	651 3 10	
Electrical and X-ray	502 2 8	
Oxygen, Stimulants, etc.	156 7 10	
Ice	8 16 0	£3,143 3 11

III. Domestic

Coal and Firewood	£1044 16 2	
Gas and Electricity	558 0 8	
Drapery, Napery, etc.	279 1 8	
Renewals and Repairs	121 13 9	
Sundries	56 19 0	
Cottage Home	241 15 1	£2,302 6 4

IV. Establishment

Renewals and repairs	£893 18 11	
Printing, Advertising, and Stationery	253 5 4	
Window Cleaning	44 12 6	
Insurance	143 15 7	
Furnishings	212 12 1	£1,548 4 5

V. Salaries and Wages

Nursing	£3087	3	4			
Medical	360	0	0			
Other Officers	300	0	0			
Dispensing and Radiology	356	0	0			
Collection	191	1	8			
Clerical	167	9	8			
Porters, Servants, &c.	2974	15	8			
Cottage Home	214	16	8	£7,651	7	0
				£18,710	11	5

B. ADMINISTRATION

I. Management

Auditor	£5	5	0			
Sanitary Inspection	4	4	0			
Flag Day Costs	86	2	4			
Legal Expenses Outlays	5	0	10	100	12	2

II. Finance (including £898 7s. 9d.
David Ferguson Trust surplus income
transferred to Building Appeal Fund)   937 17 8

C. OTHER EXPENSES

Telephone	£95	18	10			
Feuduties	25	6	0			
Rates and Taxes	115	0	5			
Sundries	136	10	5			
Cottage Home	63	15	2	436	10	10
				£20,181	12	1

D. EXTRAORDINARY EXPENDITURE

Portable X-Ray Unit	£146	10	0			
Sporoclast Dressing Sterilizer	119	7	6			
Circulating Pump Heating Apparatus ...	76	0	0			
Electrical Replacement and Repairing						
Heating Apparatus	43	4	5			
Fuel Economiser — New Pipes	24	0	0	£409	1	11
Cottage Home — New House, Builder,						
Joiner, Painter, Electrical Work,						
Furnishings				£711	6	6
				£1,120	8	5

Total Funds at close of 1936

Stocks etc... £170,324 7 1

Union Bank of Scotland Ltd.
        On Current Account   £68 19 11
        On Deposit Account 1250 0 0   1,318 19 11

Petty Cash in Matron's, etc., hands   26 0 0   £171,669 7 0

                                                                  £192,971 7 6

REFERENCES

CHAPTER 6

1.   Leith Hospital Annual Report, 1936.
2.   Leith Hospital Board of Managers, Minutes 19.10.1933.
3.   Leith Hospital Admission Book, Medical 1936.
4.   Leith Hospital Admission Book, Surgical 1936.
5.   Leith Hospital Admission Book, Children's Wing, Medical 1936.
6.   Leith Hospital Annual Report, 1946.
7.   Leith Hospital Board of Managers, Minutes 19.2.1931.
8.   Ibid., 19.2.1931.
9.   Ibid., 3.9.1942.
10. Ibid., 17.11.1938.
11. Ibid., 15.8.1935.
12. Leith Hospital Honorary Medical Staff Committee, Minutes 27.1.1935.
13. Leith Hospital Board of Managers, Minutes 20.10.1938.
14. Leith Hospital Annual Report, 1939.
15. Leith Hospital Board of Managers, Minutes 21.10.1937.
16. Leith Hospital Annual Report, 1936.
17. Leith Hospital Board of Managers, Minutes 11.2.1932.
18. Ibid., 16.6.1932.
19. Ibid., 17.4.1935.
20. Leith Hospital Annual Report, 1934
21. Ibid., 1935.
22. Leith Hospital Board of Managers, Minutes 9.3.1935.
23. Ibid., 14.5.1936.
24. Ibid., 18.3.1937.
25. Ibid., 18.11.1937.
26. Leith Hospital Annual Report, 1937.
27. Ibid., 1935.
28. Leith Hospital Board of Managers, Minutes 17.4.1935.
29. Ibid., 18.5.1939.
30. Quarterly Meeting of Royal College of Physicians of Edinburgh, Minutes July, 1975.
31. Ibid., May, 1975

32. Ibid., November, 1976.
33. *British Medical Journal* (1959), Vol. 2, p. 829.
34. *University of Edinburgh Journal* (1982), Vol. 30. p. 252.
35. Quarterly Meeting of Royal College of Physicians of Edinburgh, Minutes November, 1982.
36. *British Medical Journal* (1957), Vol. 1, p. 951.
37. Leith Hospital Board of Managers, Minutes 17.2.1938.
38. Ibid., 21.7.1939.
39. Leith Hospital Annual Report, 1912.
40. Quarterly Meeting of Royal College of Physicians of Edinburgh, Minutes May 1954.
41. *British Medical Journal* (1987), Vol. 295 p. 861.
42. Leith Hospital Board of Managers, Minutes 27.6.1934.
43. Ibid., 19.7.1934.
44. Ibid., 21.3.1935.
45. Ibid., 10.2.1938.
46. Davidson, Dr C. H., Personal Communication.
47. Leith Hospital Annual Report 1936.
48. Leith Hospital Board of Managers, Minutes 19.10.1933.
49. Ibid., 11.10.1934.
50. Leith Hospital Annual Report, 1935.
51. *The Scotsman*, 29.4.1937.
52. Leith Hospital Board of Managers, Minutes 13.5.1937.
53. Ibid., 8.7.1937.
54. Leith Hospital Annual Report, 1933.
55. Leith Hospital Board of Managers, Minutes 15.8.1935.
56. Leith Hospital Annual Report, 1938.
57. Leith Hospital Board of Managers, Minutes 16.2.1939.
58. Ibid., 13.10.1938.
59. Ibid., 27.9.1939.
60. Leith Hospital Annual Report 1939.
61. Ibid., 1940.
62. Ibid., 1940.
63. Leith Hospital Board of Managers, Minutes 9.5.1940.
64. Ibid., 1.9.1940.
65. Ibid., 20.2.1941.
66. Ibid., 15.7.1943.
67. Ibid., 20.6.1940.
68. Ibid., 19.6.1941.
69. Ibid., 16.4.1942.
70. Ibid., 8.5.1941.
71. Ibid., 19.10.1941.
72. Ibid., 19.8.1943.
73. *The Scotsman*, 6.3.1940.
74. Leith Hospital Board of Managers, Minutes 16.8.1940.
75. Ibid., 5.10.1944.
76. Leith Hospital Annual Report, 1945.
77. Leith Hospital Board of Managers, Minutes 19.10.1944.
78. Leith Hospital Annual Report, 1941.
79. Leith Hospital Board of Managers, Minutes 21.1.1943.

80.   Leith Hospital Clinical Staff Committee, Minutes 25.1.1948.
81.   Leith Hospital Annual Report, 1941.
82.   Leith Hospital Board of Managers, Minutes 7.9.1946.
83.   Ibid., 21.9.1939.
84.   Ibid., 20.6.1940.
85.   Ibid., 18.1.1940.
86.   Ibid., 11.7.1940.
87.   Ibid., 15.10.1942.
88.   Ibid., 8.1.1942.
89.   Ibid., 21.8.1941.
90.   Ibid., 9.4.1941.
91.   Ibid., 17.6.1943.
92.   Ibid., 15.8.1940.
93.   *Edinburgh Evening News* 22.1.1940.
94.   Leith Hospital Board of Managers, Minutes 17.7.1941.
95.   Ibid., 18.6.1939.
96.   Ibid., 7.12.1943.
97.   Ibid., 5.4.1945.
98.   Leith Hospital Board of Managers, Memorandum, June 1943.
99.   Leith Hospital Annual Report, 1936.
100. Leith Hospital Board of Managers, Minutes 27.3.1946.
101. Ibid., 19.12.1946.
102. Ibid., 15.5.1947.
103. Ibid., 16.5.1946.
104. Ibid., 15.5.1947.
105. Ibid., 16.12.1943.
106. Ibid., 2.10.1947.
107. Ibid., 20.1.1946.
108. Ibid., 9.5.1940.
109. Ibid., 4.10.1945.
110. Ibid., 18.9.1947.
111. Leith Hospital Annual Report, 1948.
112. Leith Hospital Board of Managers, Minutes 5.7.1945.
113. Quarterly Meeting of Royal College of Physicians of Edinburgh, Minutes, February 1972.
114. *British Journal of Urology* (1988), Vol. 62, p. 286.
115. Quarterly Meeting of Royal College of Physicians of Edinburgh, Minutes, May 1962.
116. *British Medical Journal* (1966), Vol. 2 (2), p. 1270.
117. Leith Hospital Board of Managers, Minutes 6.6.1946.
118. Leith Hospital Clinical Staff Committee, Minutes 13.1.1946.
119. Leith Hospital Board of Managers, Minutes 26.3.1947.
120. Ibid., 5.12.1946.
121. Ibid., 9.1.1947.
122. Ibid., 28.5.1948.
123. Ibid., 16.3.1944.
124. Ibid., 18.4.1946.
125. Leith Hospital Annual Report, 1948.

CHAPTER 7

The N.H.S. Established. 1948-1970

On the "appointed day" — 5th July 1948 — the Board of Managers ceased to manage and administer Leith Hospital which became one of many hospitals under the control of the South East Regional Hospital Board. The South East region included not only Edinburgh and the surrounding Lothians but parts of Fife and the Borders and administration was therefore devolved locally to Boards of Management, Leith Hospital being administered by the Board of Management for Edinburgh Northern Hospitals. The Northern Hospital Group included in addition to Leith Hospital, the Western General Hospital, Northern General Hospital, Eastern General Hospital and Musselburgh Maternity Hospital and as some of these were much larger and were to become important centres of teaching, research and specialisation, Leith eventually missed the undivided attention of its own managers. Moreover there was an increase in committee structure and thereby a certain clumsiness in administrative function; Leith matters could be discussed at the Board of Management meetings but also at the Chairman's Committee, General Purposes Committee, Finance Committee, Medical Committee and Nursing Committee and there was a small sub-committee for each of the hospitals, the first for Leith Hospital comprising Mr Ian C. Bell, Mrs Haultain and Baillie Scott.

The NHS management structure was of course in being before the appointed day, the inaugural meeting of the Board of Management Edinburgh Northern Hospitals taking place on 16th June 1948. It had twenty-four members with Professor G. A. Montgomery, KC, as chairman and Mr John Bruce, CBE, FRCSE as vice-chairman; Dr Greenlees chairman of the South East Regional Hospital Board and Dr H. A. Raeburn, senior administrative medical officer of the region, were in attendance.[1] Among the first matters of business it considered with regard to Leith Hospital were the appointment of a stores steward, the appointment of six house officers and the consideration of the building programme which included additional staff quarters above the medical wards and the reconstruction of 2-4 Mill Lane as a residency. At subsequent meetings detailed consideration was given to the provision of medical auxiliaries and administrative staff at Leith Hospital.[2] Medical auxiliaries existing and proposed were as follows:

	Present	Proposed
Pharmacist	1	1 (plus unqualified dispenser)

Physiotherapists		
Superintendents	1	1
Physiotherapists	1	2.5

Almoner	—	1

Radiographers		
Superintendent	1	1
Radiographers	1	1

Occupation therapist	—	)
Dietician	—	) Share from group
Chiropodist	—	)

The proposed administrative and service staffing was —
Hospital steward and three assistants.
Records Officer and two assistants.
Almoner's clerical assistant.
Clinical staff clerical assistants, four.
Part-time chaplain.
Telephonist/receptionist, three.
Tradesmen, seven.
Porters, eight.
Part-time hairdresser.
It was not long, however, before contentious matters surfaced.

The Problems of Endowments and Finance
At the outset the Board of Management experienced difficulties with Leith Hospital (Incorporated) which had gone into voluntary liquidation on 23rd August 1948 but still held the considerable sums of money in the hospital's endowment trusts. The smooth transfer of these funds did not take place and eventually in 1950 the Board of Management raised an action in the Court of Session. Despite what has been recorded with regard to the Leith Hospital treasurer's report in 1948 the Board of Management's accountants after examining the books and accounts of Leith Hospital for a period of ten years before the appointed day and having obtained such further evidence as they desired from the liquidators, the funds held were as follows:

1. Bed endowment	£89,833.12/- 0d.
2. Cot endowment	£13,626.15/- 8d.
3. Cottage home endowment	£1,847.18/- 11d.
4. Out-patient Department endowment	£1,069.4/- 11d.
5. Children's wing endowment	£26,708.19/- 6d.
6. Eye department endowment (Ferguson bequest)	£43,790.3/- 5d.
7. Balance of ordinary fund	£18,512.17/-6d.

and in addition —

8. Building Appeal Fund	£37,746.5/- 9d.
making a total of —	£233,135.17/- 8d.[3]

The Board of Management as pursuers asked the court to declare that prior to 5th July 1948 the property was held by the governing body of Leith Hospital solely for the purposes of the hospital and they also sued "for count, reckoning and payment" for a sum of £300,000. They argued that in terms of section 6 of the N.H.S. (Scotland) 1947 Act, the institution was transferred to the Secretary of State for Scotland and that in terms of section 7, all endowments should have been transferred to them. They had called upon the defenders to convey the property to them but they had refused or delayed to do so.

The defenders, being Leith Hospital (Incorporated) and the joint liquidators, G. A. Usher, CA and Robert Bell, WS, argued that the funds were for the carrying on of the hospital among other things and that none of the property in question was held solely for the purposes of Leith Hospital. They denied it consisted of endowments under the meaning of the Act and they went on to explain that Leith Hospital never considered that their activities were limited to the provision of hospital services. They instanced the consideration of schemes to provide a first-aid post in Leith docks, a foot clinic in Leith and financial support for convalescents and for the Samaritan Society. Particular reference was made to the Ferguson Trust of £43,790, the defender stating that in no way was it an endowment within the meaning of the Act.[4]

Evidence was given by, among others, Mr John Bruce, FRCSE, as vice-chairman of the Board of Management, Edinburgh Northern Hospitals and Mr J. H. C. A. Campbell, CA, who had examined the books of the hospital on the instructions of the solicitors for the pursuers; he had come to the conclusion that all the funds were held for the purpose of running Leith Hospital.[5] In his speech for the defenders the Dean of Faculty of Advocates, Cameron, said that there was no desire to prevent the pursuers getting that to which they were legally entitled and they were not trying to be difficult, but anxious to safeguard themselves and to obtain a judicial decision on an issue not by any means easy to solve.[6]

Lord Sorn's lengthy opinion is set out in the Supreme Court records as only one other similar case had been decided in an English court in 1950. He found on the 30th May 1951 entirely in favour of the Board of Management when after a procedure role discussion he "pronounced an interlocutor whereby he declared that the whole funds held by the defenders fell to be transferred to the pursuers".[7]

Many people saw this as a victory for an impersonal state organisation over hundreds of small and large donors who specifically

PERNICIOUS ANÆMIA

BY

LEYBOURNE STANLEY PATRICK DAVIDSON

B.A.(Camb.); M.D.; F.R.C.P.E.;

Lecturer in Systematic and in Clinical Medicine in the University of Edinburgh;
Assistant Physician to the Royal Infirmary, Edinburgh;
Formerly Assistant Physician to Leith Hospital; and
Assistant to the Professor of Bacteriology, University of Edinburgh.

AND

GEORGE LOVELL GULLAND

C.M.G.; LL.D.; M.D.; F.R.C.P.E.;

Professor Emeritus of Medicine and Clinical Medicine in the University of
Edinburgh; Consulting Physician to the Royal Infirmary, Edinburgh.

WITH APPENDIX ON DIETETIC TREATMENT
By RUTH PYBUS,
Sister Dietitian, Royal Infirmary, Edinburgh.

WITH 8 ILLUSTRATIONS AND 22 PLATES,
OF WHICH 12 ARE IN COLOUR

PLATE 14. Title-page of Davidson & Gulland's text on Pernicious Anaemia

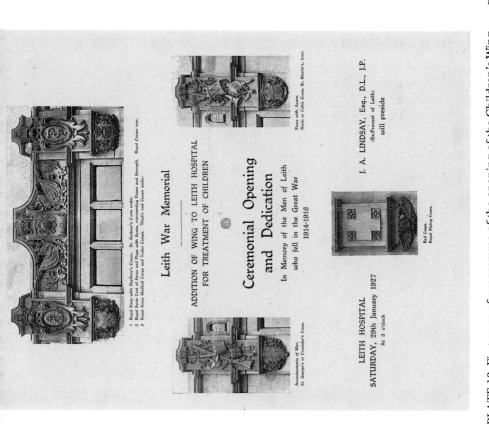

PLATE 13. First page of programme of the opening of the Children's Wing

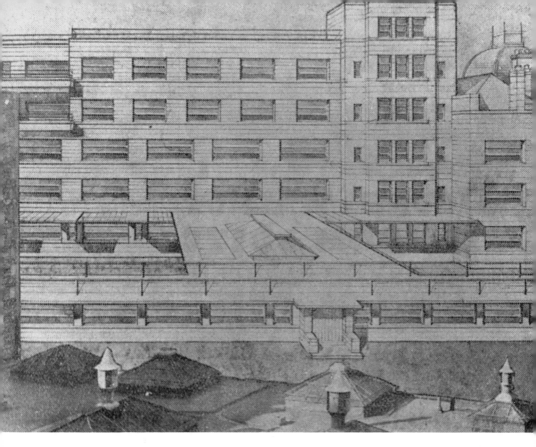

PLATE 15. Artist's impression of the proposed new medical block at Leith Hospital 1935. (By courtesy Edinburgh City Libraries)

PLATE 16. The Duke and Duchess of Kent, visiting the Children's Wing, 1935

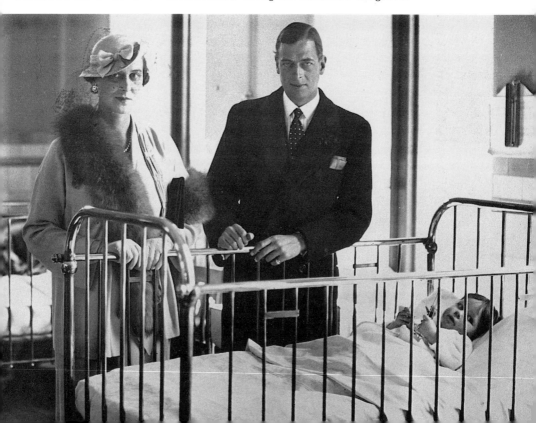

wished their gifts to benefit Leith Hospital but in the terms of the National Health Service Act the result was inevitable. There is no doubt that Leith was a relatively well off hospital in this respect and that other non-voluntary hospitals which were administered together in the Edinburgh Northern Hospital Group were sadly deprived. At the end of 1952 Leith Hospital's endowment funds were recorded at £263,527, the Northern General Hospital's at £2,126, the Western General Hospital's at £60, and the Eastern General Hospital's at £10! The balance in the Group Fund was £207.[8] This position did not however persist and Leith Hospital was not allowed to spend all the funds it once owned.

The fate of endowments was determined by a hospital Endowments Commission which was formed in 1949 and was chaired by Sir Sidney Smith, Professor of Forensic Medicine at Edinburgh University. The commission proposed a scheme for each Board of Management so that endowments might be reallocated equitably and was empowered to direct that a proportion of these be transferred to regional hospital boards and to boards of managements for hospitals with no endowments. A further power related to the allocation of endowments for medical research. The Board of Management for the Northern Hospitals was not wholly predatory in its attitude to Leith; it resolved through its finance committee that "as far as possible funds transferred . . . be earmarked for the purpose for which they were donated".[9] As a token of this the £37,000 which was in Leith's building fund was kept for building projects at Leith[10] and a liberal use was made of other funds for the purchase of a wide variety of necessary goods for the hospital. These included such diverse items as carpet-sweepers, wireless sets, dustbin trucks, steam pipes and Dunlopillow mattresses! It might be argued that money for many of these should have come from NHS funds and that other hospitals were benefiting from the release of these funds for their use. Endowment funds were even used in 1951 to combat through Pesticidal Services (Scotland) Ltd., a serious infestation of Leith Hospital by mice, rats, cockroaches and steam flies![11]

The Medical Committee of the Board of Management reviewing endowments and after a meeting with the Hospital Endowment's Commission agreed that instead of the £80,000 allocated for research purposes (representing 40 per cent of the Board's endowments) being held by the Board of Management, it should be transferred to a central body with all applications being scrutinised by a Medical Research Advisory Committee.[12] As to the other uses of these funds a scheme of allocation was eventually agreed. In 1957 sums were allotted to each hospital according to their bed complement and on the basis of £10 per bed endowment income and £5 per bed for long term equipment; so that Leith Hospital with 173 beds received £865 for equipment and £1,730 for other endowment purposes whereas the Western General Hospital with 428 beds received £2,140 and £4,280 respectively.[13] By that year also the total sum available for Leith Hospital was £53,440[14] a very considerable change in the hospital's financial fortune. The following year the board decided that the balance of endowments held and any sums received under section 58 of the Act would if not used for the specific purpose for which given in six months, be transferred to a single fund to be known as the "The Staff and Patient's Amenity Fund".[15] Only a few years later however in 1962 the consultant staff was lamenting that after alterations to the physiotherapy department were completed the monies available for building projects would be practically all used up.[16]

Donations of money and legacies continued to be made directly to Leith Hospital by patients and former patients in particular and the role of the charitable and voluntary bodies associated with the hospital is described later. It was agreed that money so given could be used "entirely at the discretion of the matron".[17] Shortly before this the General Purposes Committee had recommended that the practice at Leith of placing plaques above beds be discontinued and that donations be acknowledged by recording donor's names on a plaque in the Cowan Hall.[18]

The hospital soon found that it had not exchanged the difficulties of raising money to provide day to day running costs from voluntary services for plentiful state funds. The NHS coffers were not bottomless and as early as 1952 Leith Hospital medical staff received a letter from the treasurer of the Board of Management indicating the necessity for the saving of £10,000 in the Northern Hospital Group in the next three months.[19] In 1957-1958 however a sum of £132,000 was provided for the running costs of Leith Hospital.[20]

The Work of the Hospital after the Inauguration of the NHS

Services Lost

It became clear that with the management and administration of the hospital based on a group and ultimately a regional structure, consideration of medical services provided there was influenced by the needs of a community larger and more widely dispersed than Leith. To achieve efficiency with economy some specialties were thought to be best concentrated in fewer hospitals and from the start of the NHS therefore Leith was in danger of losing some specialist services which had been so painstakingly built up over the years.[21] As early as 1952 the consultant staff was expressing concern about the possible closure of ENT and gynaecological beds and were regretting the lack of consultation by the South East Regional Hospital Board with them.[22] The gynaecological inpatient service came to an end in the early 1950s, the speciality in the Edinburgh Northern Hospital Group being concentrated in the Western General Hospital and the Eastern General Hospital, but an outpatient clinic in gynaecology was continued at Leith and was served by consultants based at the Eastern General Hospital.

Decisions on some of these matters were slow in being made and it was not until 1966 that the ENT inpatient service was transferred to the City Hospital.[23] Objections were made even more forceably than in connection with the gynaecological beds as ENT outpatient clinics were also withdrawn shortly afterwards; representations from the medical staff warned of adverse effects on nursing training and service to patients[24] but even a last minute appeal from the Leith Hospital Committee direct to the South East Regional Hospital Board was to no avail.[25] The vacated beds were allotted to paediatric and general surgical use.[26]

Similar concerns were expressed over the proposal to withdraw ophthalmic services. Reference has already been made to the Ferguson bequest of just over £40,000 to the eye department which enabled thoughts of development in this field to be seriously contemplated at Leith Hospital. In 1956 Leith Hospital Committee in the light of a memorandum prepared by the clinical staff recommended to the regional board that an ophthalmic inpatient and outpatient department at Leith Hospital be approved and that the cost of erection and furnishing be met from endowment funds[27] but the regional board rejected this on the grounds that it was not in line with regional requirements.[28] Although the clinicians of the Edinburgh Northern Hospital Group supported the continuance of an ophthalmic outpatient department they felt unable to support an inpatient service[29] and these beds closed following Dr Leed's retiral in 1966.[30] As an example however of the uncertainties that existed in regional planning a Regional Hospital Board Planning Committee suggested in 1959 that a 40-bedded ophthalmic unit be created at Leith Hospital replacing the children's unit[31] but ophthalmology was eventually housed in the Princess Alexandra Eye Pavilion at the Edinburgh Royal Infirmary started in 1965. Former ENT and ophthalmic beds were utilised by general and paediatric surgery but an attempt to create a special care area for the hospital in one of the small vacated wards was thwarted by the Regional Hospital Board.[32]

Services Maintained, Increased and Started

The inpatient work continued to increase slightly overall with in 1966, a total of 2,651 adult patients and 1,461 children admitted (Table 8). The surgical bed complement had increased which partly accounts for the considerable increase in surgical inpatient activity and by the late 1960s the surgical unit was part of the surgical waiting day scheme involving the other acute hospitals in Edinburgh. With an unchanged bed complement medical admissions had steadily increased since before the war — achieved by a higher bed turnover. This also applied to the paediatric wards and was achieved without the convalescent facilities previously available and which by this time were inadequate.[33] Yet again, in 1968, Leith Hospital was being proposed as a suitable site for 10-12 beds for VD cases in the Edinburgh Northern Hospital area. Once again this was thought to be inappropriate.[34] The bed complements for this period were as follows: (1966 being the year ENT and ophthalmic beds were closed)

1956
ADULT   Medical — 42   CHILDREN   Medical — 20
              Surgical — 48   Surgical — 19
              (inc. ENT)   ENT   —   7
              Eyes   —   4   46
              Sick bay —   3
                               97

                                                   TOTAL— 143

1966
ADULT   Medical — 42   CHILDREN   Medical — 20
              Surgical — 74   Surgical — 16
              (inc. eyes)   ENT   —   6
              ENT   —   7   42
                           124

                                                   TOTAL— 166

Overall outpatient attendances however fell, possible explanations being the change in primary care practice following the advent of the NHS and the decline of population around the hospital, as slum property was demolished and the occupants housed in other parts of Edinburgh. An astonishing proposal was made in 1969 in a letter from the Group Medical Superintendent that outpatient services at Leith Hospital be withdrawn altogether, the object being to increase the utilisation of the newly opened outpatient department at the Western General Hospital![35] This was vigorously rejected by the clinical staff of Leith Hospital and received no firm backing from other bodies.

One outpatient service was added in this time — a psychiatric clinic which in 1966 dealt with forty-one new patients and was conducted by Dr Lassalle based at the Royal Edinburgh Hospital.[36]

The arrangements for laboratory work before the NHS has been described. The laboratory of the Royal College of Physicians of Edinburgh closed in 1950 and in any event, after 1948 the Board of Management, Edinburgh Northern Hospitals, organised laboratory services for all the hospitals in the Group. Bacteriological services were based at the Northern General Hospital under the direction of Dr McCabe and Dr Nancy Conn and later were based at the new central microbiological laboratory at the Western General Hospital under Dr Gould. Biochemistry was also initially based at the Northern General Hospital and then at the Western General Hospital. Pathology and histology were centred at the Western General Hospital, the consultant pathologist there contributing a more direct service to Leith Hospital by continuing to perform post-mortem examinations at the hospital's own post-mortem room. Although these laboratories were not on the hospital premises Leith Hospital did not have a poorer service than before but indeed enjoyed an enhanced service as an efficient organisation of vans operated between all the hospitals of the group and the laboratories. House physicians were able to time the taking of specimens to catch several upliftings during the day and outwith normal hours taxis were used to take urgent specimens rapidly for examination.

One important area of work which in earlier days was covered by nursing and medical staff and was now run by an efficient and professional ancillary service was dietetics, although Leith in the early days was insufficiently served in this respect. Before 1957 a dietician from the Western General Hospital provided a limited outpatient service to Leith Hospital. In that year a dietician was appointed to the Eastern General Hospital and she provided a necessary limited service to Leith Hospital.[37] Not surprisingly it was the paediatricians who found this restriction most irkesome and in 1964 Dr Keay, consultant paediatrician, pointed out that such disorders as coeliac disease and phenylketonuria could not be properly treated in the hospital because of this deficiency.[38] In due course a more liberal allocation of dietician sessions was provided for Leith Hospital these being the basis of the very satisfactory service it enjoyed latterly from these health professionals, a service which will be referred to later.

The casualty department at the hospital first came under threat in the 60s. There was a view that casualty services in the City should be concentrated in the Royal Infirmary of Edinburgh and the Western General Hospital. In 1964 however the Regional Hospital Board published a statement of policy retaining the casualty department at Leith but grading it as a peripheral accident unit.[39] Unease amongst medical and surgical staff and others persisted at the hospital and was expressed in 1968 when it was thought that the opening of the new department at the Western General Hospital would result in the closure of the Leith department. Reassurance came from the medical superintendent who assured the staff that it would still be necessary to maintain a peripheral accident service at Leith.[40]

Some idea of new concepts in the practice of medicine in the hospital come from the minutes of the Clinical Staff Meetings, one in 1961 being a reflection on early methods of resuscitation in cardiac arrest.[41] In a discussion on equipment required, "simple equipment for opening the chest" was thought necessary but a rider was added that this equipment, though, advantageous was costly and should not prejudice the purchase of other more necessary equipment! Later that year a defibrillator was purchased for the hospital.

The main clinical work of the hospital was carried out by generalists of a high calibre and wide experience but was not of a type to figure frequently in the medical literature. In 1960 however circumstances arose which are recorded by Catford in his book *"The Royal Infirmary of Edinburgh 1929-1979"* but which by right have a place in the history of Leith Hospital as well. Dr R. F. Robertson one of Leith's two consultant physicians at that time had a patient attending the hospital with severe renal disease which ultimately resulted in chronic renal failure. Learning that the patient had a healthy identical twin, Dr Robertson very astutely realised that a renal transplant was possible. The patient was admitted to the Edinburgh Royal Infirmary where the first successful transplant of a human kidney was performed in the United Kingdom. The transplant was performed on 30th October 1960 by Professor Woodruff but the operation on the donor was performed by Mr J. A. Ross, a consultant surgeon at Leith Hospital. Leith therefore had cause to be proud of its association with this milestone in the treatment of renal disease.

Lastly a curious footnote to a practice which had been accepted for decades at the hospital comes in the minutes of the Board of Management for 1960. It is to the effect that the custom of putting up a list at the main entrance of the names of dangerously ill patients in the hospital should be discontinued![42]

Building Development at the Hospital

The last major construction work at Leith was the children's wing in the 1920s and the new nurses home in the 1930s and 40s but the managers had had plans for further development which as has been recounted did not take place. During the war little had been done to improve the fabric of the building and the memory of one physician who joined the staff after the war is somewhat depressing. The medical wards were painted a universal brown typical of 19th century institutional decor; there was no bed lift to the medical wards patients being carried upstairs on stretchers; there was no appointment system and patients waited sometimes for hours on hard benches in the Cowan Hall to be seen in an inadequate outpatient department.[43] Three years after the start of the NHS in 1951 the clinical staff was moved to deplore the deterioration of the fabric of the hospital since nationalisation.[44]

In the first few months of the NHS it was still the intention of the Board of Management to proceed with the reconstruction of number 2-4 Mill Lane as a residency. This intention was soon abandoned when the pressing need for a new outpatient department became clear and in 1951 these premises were opened for outpatient purposes, a function which they still fulfil.[45] Although a great improvement on previous facilities it was far from ideal as outpatients requiring for example, x-ray examinations had to cross a public thoroughfare to the main hospital. This serious drawback prompted the General Purposes Committee of the Board of Management to make an application to the authorities to close Mill Lane entirely at least to heavy traffic (as had been done earlier with regard to King Street) but to no avail.[46]

A number of alterations and upgradings were carried out in the two decades after nationalisation. Piecemeal, they were not immediately impressive in extent but they are seen as a whole in an article which appeared in the *Edinburgh Evening News* in 1964 under the headline "£110,000 Conversion at Leith Hospital".[47] This described a major scheme of reconstruction which had been completed after eight years of work and included the conversion of two wards (5 and 6) into a single u-shaped ward of thirty beds, a piped oxygen supply and, at last, a lift to service the medical wards. During the work carried out on the last item it was found that a section of hospital foundations (the original 1848-50 building) appeared to be on sand and it had to be redesigned.[48] The newspaper report went on to describe facilities provided to allow Leith Hospital to be among the first to offer a choice of meals to patients. This was associated with a waitress service for patients instituted on an experimental basis at the request of the Scottish Home and Health Department[49] and which was said two years later to be a success.[50] Most of the £110,000 came from endowments, by then under the control of the Edinburgh Northern Hospitals Board of Management; the tax-payer, the newspaper pointed out, contributed only £40,000! It was also stressed that it was unusual for an entire hospital to be converted out of free funds.

Despite all this there were difficulties. The clinical staff noted with great relief the date of reopening of the main surgical theatre after reconstruction (26th November 1956), sixteen months after closure![51] Moreover clinical staff considered in 1960 that the Board of Management was inhibited in carrying out more expensive upgrading in view of the uncertain function of Leith Hospital in future plans of the Regional Hospital Board. On the other hand Dr Forfar, consultant paediatrician, proposed a party to celebrate the completion of upgrading in the children's wing in 1960, alterations which resulted in a medical bed complement of twenty but a reduction in surgical beds from twenty-six to twenty-two.[52]

Alterations in the x-ray department in 1956 were necessary because of a report by the group senior physicist who found that although none of the radiographers received a dose of radiation in excess of the maximum permissible, they recorded a dose five to ten times higher than staff at the Western General Hospital.[53]

In the 1960s as will be described later there was increase in the medical teaching activity in the hospital and alterations and upgrading of premises were necessary to cope with this. The University and the Regional Board undertook joint responsibility for improvements to a teaching room and a student's common room to the tune of £250 and £500 respectively and £100 was allotted from a Group endowment to start a medical reference library.[54]

Finally it was at this time (1961-62) that a yard next to the outpatient department was laid out as a rose garden for the benefit of patients and staff.[55]

Nursing and the Demise of Nursing Training at the Hospital

The survival of an independent school of nursing at Leith was in doubt from the beginning of the NHS, a suggestion that the Western General Hospital, Northern General Hospital and Leith Hospital should form a group for nurse training being made in 1949.[56] In 1951 a bus was being provided to convey nurses from Leith to the preliminary training school at the Western General Hospital[57] and later the same year the Nursing Committee was debating the difficulty experienced by Leith Hospital in recruiting sufficient nurses.[58] A brochure for the recruitment of nurses at Leith was produced in 1952 and the Nursing Committee requested the matron at the Western General Hospital to refer any applicants who could not be employed there to Leith.[59] Three years later Leith failed to attract a suitable candidate for the post of sister tutor and it was recommended that the post be re-advertised stressing participation in teaching at the school at the Western General.[60] In 1958 a letter was received from the Secretary of the Regional Nurse Training Committee alleging that requirements for general training were not being wholly fulfilled at Leith, an allegation that was rejected by the hospital.[61] Another indication of erosion of enthusiasm for training at Leith was the cancellation for two years running in the late 50s of the nurses prize giving, a circumstance which was deplored by the medical staff who debated how help could be given to the matron in her difficulties.[62]

Altogether the writing was on the wall as regards nurse training at Leith and in 1969 it was recorded that the final six nursing students in training had now completed that training and that henceforth this would be the function entirely of the North Edinburgh School of Nursing.[63] No longer therefore did nurses accept with pride their certificate (an example of which is seen in plate 17) at the end of their training at Leith Hospital. Thus came to an end an excellent small school which it may be argued existed from the time probationers were first accepted in 1875. However there exists a copy of the brochure mentioned above which has a surprising statement on the cover, the words "Founded AD 1837". This is certainly a mistake as formal nursing training was not started even in the Royal Infirmary of Edinburgh until the 1860s. It is just possible of course that the date refers to the founding of the hospital rather than the School of Nursing but even then it anticipates by more than a decade.

Miss McKee who had been appointed matron in 1943 retired with the advent of the NHS in 1948 and was replaced by Miss McGregor Mitchell. She served for eighteen years until 1966 when Miss Beale took up the post. Miss Mitchell had the responsibility for the nursing care of patients in 170 beds or cots. To carry this out she had a larger staff than had existed before but even more nurses were proposed in a 1949 review of nursing establishment[64] details of which are as follows:

	ACTUAL	PROPOSED
Matron	1	1
Assistant Matron	1	1
Departmental sister	0	1
Home sister	1	1
Assistant home sister	1	0
Night superintendent	1	1
Sister tutor (S)	1	1
Sister tutor (A)	1	1
Theatre sisters	2	2
Ward sisters	7	8
Night sister	1	1
Staff nurses	14	18
Student nurses	69	90
Male theatre orderly	1	1
	100	117

From what has been said about the School of Nursing, its difficulties of recruitment and demise, it is not surprising that the ideal proved impossible to obtain.

Another sign of the times in the 1960s was the beneficiary of a dance organised by student nurses at the hospital in Leith Town Hall. In previous times the financial gains from such an enterprise would have without question gone to the hospital for its sole benefit but in 1966 the £50 raised went to the Marie Curie Foundation.[65]

Medical staffing after 1948

Senior medical staff were appointed as NHS consultants but their employing authority was the South East Regional Hospital Board and they were appointed to one of the hospital groups and had varying numbers of sessions at individual hospitals. At Leith Hospital few had all their sessions there. Junior hospital staff on the other hand were largely appointed to the individual units of the hospital with the exception of some paediatric and anaesthetic staff who had commitments at the Western General Hospital or others or who rotated through different units.

Subtle and sometimes not so subtle changes took place in the practice and attitudes of medical staff. In February 1949 it was suggested at a meeting of the clinical staff of the hospital that now they were members of the Northern Hospital Group staff there was little need for separate meetings of Leith staff but it was agreed to continue with extraordinary meetings when required.[66] In fact Leith Hospital Clinical Staff Committee continued to function until the closure of the hospital. Consultants were charged for meals taken in the residency[67] and one of the first casualties of house officers' perquisites at Leith Hospital was the General Purpose Committee's discontinuance of the supply of beer![68] Not all was lost however as the Medical Committee noted at the end of 1948 that house officers at the former municipal hospitals were paid £120 for their six month service whereas house officers at Leith received £80;[69] a uniform rate of £120 plus emoluments was agreed. One "perk" which was not denied to house officers was free entry to the Eldorado Stadium which by that time housed all-in wrestling. There, such fierce combatants as "Rough-house" Baker, Jack Pye and his brother "Dirty" Pye did battle.[70] It is curious that medical staff who remember the violence of these bouts are all agreed that they never saw injuries resulting from them.[71] In contrast to this when many years later in the late 1970s the stadium had a brief life as a skateboard arena, the casualty staff saw many youngsters with a variety of injuries.

The practice of appointing "consulting" physicians or surgeons as a way of doing honour to individuals lapsed with the NHS although there is an exception to this, namely, the appointment of Mr J. R. Cameron as consulting surgeon in 1967. Following active service with the RAMC in the second world war he served as surgeon to the hospital (having previously been assistant surgeon) from 1947-54 moving at that time to the Edinburgh Royal Infirmary and later to become President of the Royal College of Surgeons of Edinburgh. He was an accomplished endocrine surgeon and made a reputation for his skill in the surgery of malignant melanoma, sometimes making reference in a self-deprecatory way to the "mole-catcher". Mr David Band was surgeon to the hospital for a brief period from 1944-1947 before taking charge of the urological department at the Western General Hospital. After the war a number of surgeons were appointed some of whom had been assistant surgeons in the past. J. A. Ross had a distinguished career in the RAMC which brought the reward of an MBE and which he has recounted in his book *"Memoirs of an Army Surgeon"*. He moved to the surgical unit of the Eastern General Hospital in 1961 and later he also became a President of the Royal College of Surgeons of Edinburgh. T. I. (Tammas) Wilson served Leith from 1949.

Thomas Ian Wilson (1910-1983). Graduating MB in 1933 and obtaining the FRCSE in 1937 he worked both with Sir David Wilkie and Sir Henry Wade. After war service in India and Burma he was on the staff of Edinburgh Royal Infirmary and Leith Hospital until 1967 when he took on the task of setting up a new urological department in the Infirmary. He was a councillor of the RCSE for fifteen years.[72]

Arthur Fawcett Miller Barron, VRD, OBE (1912-1971) graduated MB at Edinburgh in 1935, MD with commendation in 1938 and became an FRCSE in 1939. He served with distinction in the RNVR throughout the war and later continued his naval connection being principle medical officer to the Forth Division RNVR with the rank of surgeon commander from 1946-1958. Just after the war he was clinical tutor to Mr Jardine at Edinburgh Royal Infirmary and then surgeon to Leith Hospital. From 1955-1967 he also had sessions at Longmore Hospital. He was instrumental in encouraging the development of Leith Hospital as a full under-graduate teaching unit. He had a lasting love of the sea and was a member of the Royal Forth Yacht Club.[73]

Donald MacKintosh moved to Edinburgh Royal Infirmary in 1954. Following his war service he became known as an expert in the surgery of the thyroid gland.

In the 50s W. P. Small joined the staff before becoming surgeon to the gastrointestinal unit at the Western General Hospital and Eric Gilmour was appointed surgeon until his retirement in 1978. He had served with the first army in North Africa and Europe and was surgeon at the Deaconess Hospital as well as Leith. The carparks of both hospitals achieved an air of elegance when his stately grey Rolls-Royce was present. In the 60s John Cook and Archibald McPherson were appointed. Archie McPherson was renowned for his surgery of portal hypertension and the spleen and for peripheral vascular surgery; John Cook had been a senior lecturer at Makerere University where his work on Kaposi's sarcoma became very well known and he later became surgeon at the Eastern General Hospital and Secretary and Vice-President of the Royal College of Surgeons of Edinburgh. The paediatric surgeons appointed were Mr Robarts, Mr Ian Kirkland and Mr Bisset. Dr J. A. Bruce left Leith Hospital in 1950 to become physician at the Eastern General Hospital and Roodlands Hospital and R. M. Murray Lyon also left that year to become physician at the Edinburgh Royal Infirmary.

Ronald Malcolm Murray-Lyon (1904-1969) was the son of Thomas Murray-Lyon MD and the cousin of David Murray-Lyon professor of therapeutics at Edinburgh University. After the war in which he had served in the RAMC in hospitals in Northern Ireland, West Africa, North West Europe and India he was briefly physician at Leith Hospital and then physician at the Edinburgh Royal Infirmary. He became chief medical officer of the Life Association of Scotland.[74]

Dr Chalmers Davidson joined the staff as consultant physician in 1950 leaving in 1970 on his retirement; he was also physician to Chalmers Hospital and was honorary librarian of the Royal College of Physicians of Edinburgh for many years reflecting his deserved reputation as a bibliophile.

In 1959 he was joined by Dr R. F. Robertson who later became President of the Royal College of Physicians of Edinburgh, physician to the Queen in Scotland, President of the British Medical Association and physician to Edinburgh Royal Infirmary; he was awarded CBE in 1980. Dr J. O. Forfar M.C. was appointed paediatric physician in 1953 leaving in 1964 on his acceptance of the chair of paediatrics at Edinburgh University. Dr A. J. Keay, Secretary and Treasurer of the Royal College of Physicians of Edinburgh and Dr James Syme, also Secretary and subsequently Vice-President of the College, became paediatricians in the 60s and 70s.

Dr C. R. D. Leeds was appointed ophthalmic surgeon just before the NHS and continued in this post until 1965. Dr G. S. Dhillon also served in this capacity and was followed in the 60s by Dr Hughes who was still in post on the closure of the hospital. From 1948 to the cessation of ENT work in the hospital C. E. Scott, A. B. Smith, F. Birrell and A. McCallum were consultants in this discipline. Immediately after the war Dr K. Herdman joined as anaesthetist and was succeeded by Dr Leslie Morrison MC. After his distinguished war service, Leslie Morrison gave unstinted and long service to Leith Hospital until his retiral in 1985. Dr Grant Peterkin was succeeded as dermatologist by Dr George Beveridge. After W. A. Liston's death and A. F. Anderson's retirement

TABLE 8

Inpatient and Outpatient Statistics 1956 and 1966

	1956		1966	
INPATIENTS	ADULT	PAEDIATRIC	ADULT	PAEDIATRIC
Surgical	1002	594	1583	754
Medical	629	294	854	548
Ophthalmic	105	9	10	6
Ear, nose and throat	192	232	204	154
	1928	1129	2651	1462
OUTPATIENTS				
Surgical	2781	307	1585	224
Medical	1170	258	905	218
Gynaecological	318	—	491	—
Ophthalmic	*1044	—	*719	—
E.N.T.	808	523	660	408
Dermatological	*951	—	*831	—
Psychiatric	—	—	41	—
Physiotherapy	*1288	1088	*1178	1269
	8360	1976	6410	2119
X-ray Department (number of patients)	*9927		+3644	
Casualty Department	*11205		*12405	

* Includes children
\+ New patients only

In 1956 — total of 49,889 return patients and in 1966 — 31,134.

the gynaecological outpatient service was continued by Dr John Loudon who served until his retirement in 1987.

In 1968 Dr Martin Fraser succeeded Dr J. G. Kinninmonth as radiologist. Kinninmonth, appointed in 1937 was one of the longest serving of Leith Hospital's consultant staff and in his later years his reports were models of clarity and brevity as Mr James Ross recalls. "On one occasion I had a case of a badly fractured tibia and fibula. X-ray report, 'Frct. Tibia in bad position'. After manipulation the x-ray report came, 'No better'. So I manipulated again and re x-rayed. This time the report came, a single word, 'Worse'. He would occasionally give credit where credit was due with the single report 'Better'."[75]

On the administrative side the first and last medical superintendent of Leith Hospital demitted office in 1948. After the NHS, a group superintendent and deputy superintendent were appointed. Dr A. B. Donald took particular responsibility for the Western General Hospital and his deputy Dr George Vaughan for the Eastern General Hospital and Leith.

REFERENCES

CHAPTER 7

1.   Edinburgh Northern Hospitals, Board of Management, Minutes 16.6.1948.
2.   Ibid., 18.10.1948. et. seq.
3.   Supreme Court Cases (1951) pp. 524-530.
4.   The Scotsman, 3.6.1950.
5.   Ibid., 9.5.1951.
6.   Ibid., 10.5.1951.
7.   Supreme Court Cases. Ibid., p. 525.
8.   Edinburgh Northern Hospitals, Board of Management, Minutes 28.1.1953.
9.   Ibid., 27.6.1951.
10.   Ibid., 18.5.1955.
11.   Ibid., 18.4.1951.
12.   Ibid., 14.11.1951.
13.   Ibid., 20.6.1957.
14.   Ibid., 9.4.1957.
15.   Ibid., 13.5.1958.
16.   Ibid., 18.7.1962.
17.   Ibid., 20.7.1955.
18.   Ibid., 21.1.1953.
19.   Leith Hospital Clinical Staff Committee, Minutes 11.1.1952.
20.   Edinburgh Northern Hospitals, Board of Management, Minutes 14.5.1957.
21.   Leith Hospital Clinical Staff Committee, Minutes 11.1.1925.
22.   Ibid., 4.12.1953.
23.   Edinburgh Northern Hospitals, Board of Management, Minutes 2.10.1966.
24.   Leith Hospital Clinical Staff Committee, Minutes 14.11.1964.
25.   Edinburgh Northern Hospitals, Board of Management, Minutes 20.4.1965.

26. Ibid., 20.4.1965.
27. Ibid., 11.12.1956.
28. Ibid., 12.3.1957.
29. Ibid., 8.7.1958.
30. Leith Hospital Clinical Staff Committee, Minutes 15.3.1965.
31. Ibid., 2.7.1959.
32. Ibid., 10.10.1967.
33. Ibid., 2.7.1959.
34. Edinburgh Northern Hospitals, Board of Management, Minutes 6.1968.
35. Leith Hospital Clinical Staff Committee, Minutes 30.1.1969.
36. Ibid., 15.3.1965.
37. Steven, Miss Fiona, Personal Communication.
38. Leith Hospital Clinical Staff Committee, Minutes 25.5.1964.
39. Edinburgh Northern Hospitals, Board of Management, Minutes 17.11.1964.
40. Ibid., 25.5.1968.
41. Leith Hospital Clinical Staff Committee, Minutes 7.7.1961.
42. Edinburgh Northern Hospitals, Board of Management, Minutes 11.10.1960.
43. Davidson, Dr C. H., Personal Communication.
44. Leith Hospital Clinical Staff Committee, Minutes 7.7.1951.
45. Ibid., 11.1.1951.
46. Edinburgh Northern Hospitals, Board of Management, Minutes 21.12.1955.
47. *Edinburgh Evening News*, 2.6.1964.
48. Edinburgh Northern Hospitals, Board of Management, Minutes 15.2.1956.
49. Ibid., 21.11.1964.
50. Ibid., 12.7.1966.
51. Leith Hospital Clinical Staff Committee, Minutes 15.11.1956.
52. Ibid., 13.12.1960.
53. Edinburgh Northern Hospitals, Board of Management, Minutes 11.12.1956.
54. Ibid., 17.10.1967.
55. Leith Hospital Clinical Staff Committee, Minutes 18.7.1962.
56. Edinburgh Northern Hospitals, Board of Management, Minutes 12.1949.
57. Ibid., 20.6.1951.
58. Ibid., 17.10.1951.
59. Ibid., 23.1.1952.
60. Ibid., 21.9.1955.
61. Ibid., 9.10.1958.
62. Leith Hospital Clinical Staff Committee, Minutes 17.2.1959.
63. Edinburgh Northern Hospitals, Board of Management, Minutes 15.7.1969.
64. Ibid., Memorandum 1949.
65. Ibid., 19.4.1966.
66. Leith Hospital Clinical Staff Committee, Minutes 3.2.1949.
67. Ibid., 16.2.1950.
68. Edinburgh Northern Hospitals, Board of Management, Minutes 3.2.1949.
69. Ibid., 18.10.1948.
70. Davidson, Dr C. H., Personal Communication.
71. Ross, Mr J. A., Personal Communication.
72. *British Medical Journal* (1983), Vol. 286, p. 1586.
73. Ibid., (1971), Vol. 3, p. 193.
74. Ibid., (1969), Vol. 1, p. 648.
75. Ross, Mr J. A., Personal Communication.

CHAPTER 8

Leith as a Teaching Hospital

The important role of Leith Hospital in the clinical teaching of women medical undergraduates in the 1880s and 1890s and in the functioning of Dr Jex Blake's Edinburgh School of Medicine for Women has already been described. Formal teaching of undergraduates ceased in 1893 and did not restart on a regular basis until the 1960s.

Nevertheless the hospital did not become a complete stranger to clinical teaching. It seems likely that individual members of the visiting staff made arrangements for clinical teaching of students at their own outpatient clinics or in their wards and certainly the medical staff expressed the desire to do so, only three years after the unfortunate rift with Dr Jex Blake.[1] When in 1898 the appointment of successors to the first gynaecologist was being discussed it was agreed they should have the right to have classes of students at the hospital.[2] In 1908 correspondence with the Clerk to the Faculty of Medicine of the University resulted in agreement that a "certificate of dressing" from the outpatient department of the hospital would be accepted by the university. The managers made the proviso that not more than six students would attend at a time and the fee was fixed at two guineas per six months attendance.[3]

A further and very unusual teaching commitment was accepted by the staff of Leith Hospital in the early part of this century. Leith Nautical College had been established in 1903 as a successor to the Leith Navigation School and was concerned with all aspects of training for ship's officers.[4] In 1904 the hospital was approached to provide demonstrations and instruction to the students in elementary surgery, medicine and hygiene.[5] This task was accepted and continued for many years. Even after he retired as physician in 1910 Dr Langwill continued his course of lectures to these future ship's officers and masters.[6]

Post-Graduate Teaching and the Proposed Post-Graduate Hospital

It was in the field of post-graduate teaching that Leith Hospital was most active in the first half of this century. As early as 1906 an approach was made from the secretary of the Edinburgh Post-Graduate Executive Committee for teaching facilities in the hospital — a request which was readily granted.[7] Thereafter there were repeated requests for renewal of these facilities from such luminaries as Professor Cunningham[8] and Professor Harvey Littlejohn[9] who were successively associated with the Post Graduate Committee. Another approach that was made in 1906 was from Sir Thomas Fraser requesting that students

of tropical diseases studying at Edinburgh University and the Edinburgh Medical School should be granted demonstrations of clinical
cases at the hospital. It was pointed out that not a large number of
patients with tropical diseases were seen at Edinburgh but that ships
arriving at Leith from all parts of the world might bring in a more
bountiful harvest! This was agreed and precise times for demonstrations arranged.[10]

The two world wars inevitably saw a temporary decline in post graduate teaching but towards the end of the second world war in 1943 the
old Post-graduate Executive Committee was succeeded by the Joint
Committee on Post-Graduate Teaching. This committee was clearly
concerned firstly with the short term problem of doctors returning
from active service with the armed forces and requiring refresher
courses and secondly the long term problem of higher professional
training. At its first meeting in December 1943 Professor Sidney Smith
of the Department of Forensic Medicine and Dean of the Faculty of
Medicine referred to the probability that a separate hospital for post-
graduate teaching would be required and that special arrangements
would have to be made for staff.[11] Recognising that it would be difficult
to find a suitable hospital within reasonable distance of the medical
school a sub-committee consisting of Professor L. S. P. Davidson of the
Chair of Medicine and former assistant physician at Leith Hospital,
Professor Murray Lyon of the Chair of Clinical Medicine and Mr Paterson Brown, surgeon at the Royal Infirmary of Edinburgh was formed
to investigate and in particular to consider the Edinburgh Municipal
Hospitals and Leith Hospital.[12] By February 1944 reports were submitted on visits paid to these hospitals. The President of the Board of
Managers of Leith Hospital, Sir Gilbert Archer, had made no secret of
his personal wish that use should be made of the hospital for medical
teaching. However, Professor Davidson reported that the medical
wards were unsuitable for teaching and side room accommodation was
inadequate. Mr Paterson Brown thought the surgical wards better than
the medical wards and although the operating theatres were good they
were not suitable for teaching; moreover side rooms were limited and
outpatient arrangements unsuitable. However as a rider to this apparently damning report it was stated that certain of the defects noted
might without much difficulty be remedied![13] There were difficulties
also with the municipal hospitals and discussion at one point swung to
consider the building of a new 200-bedded hospital for post-graduate
purposes. Yet by March of that year the committee's view was that
outwith the Royal Infirmary of Edinburgh "Leith Hospital would seem
to be the most suitable for the purpose".[14] By this time the Edinburgh
Post-Graduate Board for Medicine, its governing body consisting of
equal representation from the University of Edinburgh, the Royal College of Physicians of Edinburgh and the Royal College of Surgeons of
Edinburgh, had been formed and it had appointed a committee to

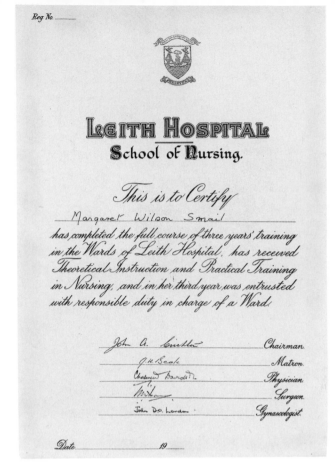

PLATE 17. Leith Hospital School of Nursing certificate, circa 1966

PLATE 18. The winning tickets in the raffle and the newly purchased ultra-sound machine are displayed. From left to right: Jim Calder, Scottish Rugby internationalist, Hector Lambie, one of the sponsors, Russell Hunter, actor, Dr Denning, Chairman of the Lothian Health Board, Dr Douglas Grieve, consultant radiologist and Mr Ian McIntyre, consultant surgeon.

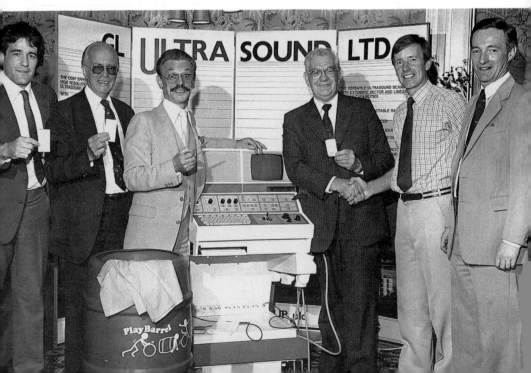

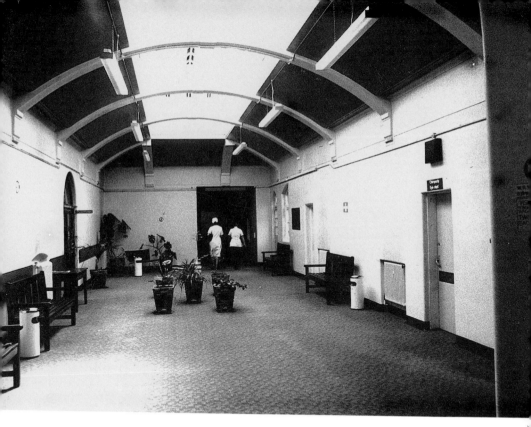

PLATE 19. The Cowan Hall in the 1980s

PLATE 20. The Red Court, reconstructed after the fire

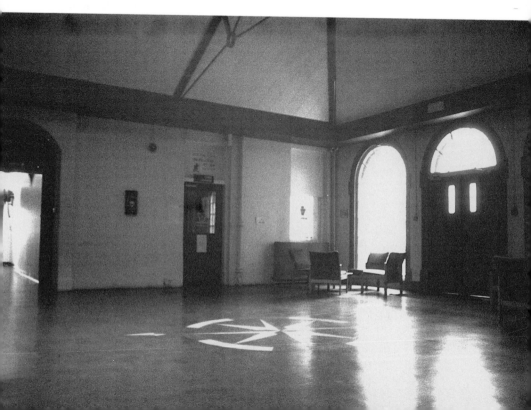

approach the Board of Management of Leith Hospital with a view to using it for post-graduate teaching.[15] In June 1945 Professor Mackie of the Department of Bacteriology and Dr C. P. Stewart of the Department of Clinical Chemistry visited Leith Hospital in connection with laboratory accommodation. Plans were submitted regarding reconstruction of rooms for this purpose.[16]

It seemed at that time that negotiations were proceeding satisfactorily but in December 1945 the Chairman of the Post-graduate Board, Professor R. N. Johnstone (who had also met Sir Gilbert Archer) had to inform his board that a considerable amount of adverse criticism had been expressed by the Leith Hospital medical staff of the proposals which had been put to them by the hospital managers.[17] The views of the honorary medical staff were that Leith Hospital was too small for sustained clinical teaching and that it lacked suitable clinical material. The staff was also concerned about the people of Leith who, it was thought, would be deprived of admission should they, when ill, be considered unsuitable clinical cases for a teaching hospital. However valid these arguments were there is determination in the recorded statement that "the staff are not prepared to resign their appointments in furtherance of an inadequate scheme of post graduate teaching in this hospital".[18]

The Post-graduate Board agreed that before further progress could be made it would be necessary to get from Leith Hospital definite acceptance of their willingness to accept the board's nominees for teaching, that those appointed would be given full charge of beds and all reasonable rights regarding the admission of patients. "Without this the scheme could not be carried out."[19] A further meeting of representatives of the Post-graduate Board with the managers of Leith Hospital at which delegates of the medical staff were present did not help. The managers felt they could not accept the proposals meantime until they had had an opportunity to study the report of the regional hospital survey and perhaps more significantly the medical staff were clearly concerned about the Post-graduate Board's insistance on nominating teaching staff. On this the Post-graduate Board decided to inform the managers that it greatly regretted their decision; acceptance of their proposals would have, they thought, not only furthered the interests of the Edinburgh Medical School, but would have been to the benefit of the hospital and the people of Leith.[20]

Thus ended an episode that had proved frustrating for all. Leith missed the opportunity of becoming perhaps the Hammersmith of Edinburgh and Edinburgh still lacks a hospital devoted to post graduate teaching and research.

Despite this the hospital continued to take a regular and active part in the courses organised by the Post-graduate Board for Medicine particularly the very popular internal medicine course and its associated clinical courses. Few weeks passed without groups of young post-graduates from all over the world being taught in medicine, surgery and paediatrics and this ceased only with the closure of the hospital. In like manner general practitioners were not strangers to Leith Hospital coming as they did as part of the refresher courses organised by the board.

Under-Graduate Teaching and Association with the University
Between and during the wars under-graduate clinical teaching in Edinburgh was largely concentrated in the Royal Infirmary. It was Sir Stanley Davidson, Professor of Medicine at Edinburgh from 1938 who was given the task immediately after the second world war of raising the standard and status of the municipal hospitals of Edinburgh, namely the Western, Northern and Eastern General Hospitals. As Sir Stanley pointed out these hospitals had been used for many years as institutions where those suffering from old age or incurable diseases were sent after they had been discharged from the Royal Infirmary or any of the other small voluntary hospitals where most of the clinical talent and modern equipment was concentrated.[21] Not surprisingly these three hospitals were not highly regarded by the public. He himself tells of an instance when he was assistant physician at Leith Hospital of overhearing a mother say to her misbehaving child, "Noo Tommy if ye dinnae behave yersel I'll pit ye tae the Eastern!"

History records how spectacularly successful Sir Stanley was in attracting first class clinicians and research workers to these hospitals and how successful the various medical units in them became. Inevitably under-graduate and post-graduate teaching was attracted to these units relieving the gross overcrowding of teaching facilities at the Royal Infirmary, and Leith Hospital shared in this decentralisation. From the mid 1960s regular under-graduate teaching was taking place at the hospital although in 1957 the Board of Studies of the Faculty of Medicine of Edinburgh University indicated the wish to include Leith Hospital for the training of five or six students in casualty work for two weeks during the term, a wish which was agreed to.[22] In 1964, again at the request of the Faculty of Medicine, resident medical students were accommodated at the hospital[23] and later that year the designation of Leith Hospital in some statistical statements as a "non-teaching hospital" was challenged as it was averred that it performed the same teaching duties as the Western General Hospital and the Eastern General Hospital which were designated as teaching hospitals.[24] As a consequence, in the 1964-65 Edinburgh University calendar, Leith was first listed as a teaching hospital and physicians, surgeons, anaesthetists, ophthalmologists and radiologists named as clinical teachers. Under-graduate teaching was securely established and of such a volume that in 1967 improvements to the teaching room and students' common room attracted grants of money from the University and Regional Hospital

Board.[25] Final phase students attended from 1970.[26] With the introduction of the new curriculum for the degrees of MB, ChB in 1978, Phase I, Phase II and Phase III students were being catered for. Phase I students (years one and two) were introduced to clinical medicine and ward routine in groups of fourteen or more. Phase II students (year three) were taught the techniques of history taking and physical examination throughout the university session and Phase III students (years four and five) spent six weeks singly or in pairs working as clinical clerks in the wards. It was from these students that most of Leith Hospital's house officers were drawn. Teaching at Leith Hospital in medicine, surgery and paediatrics proved highly popular with students.

For many years also the teaching of clinical medicine to students of the School of Dental Surgery within the Faculty of Medicine of the University of Edinburgh were taught at Leith Hospital. This task was first accepted in 1950 and intermittently thereafter.

The staff who taught these students were for the most part NHS consultants. A few were university staff with honorary consultant posts or were part time senior lecturers. The NHS staff were accorded clinical teaching staff status or were appointed honorary senior lecturers. Some had direct links with the Department of Surgery, University of Edinburgh or with the Department of Medicine, University of Edinburgh, based at the Western General Hospital. Mention must also be made of the contribution to teaching made by NHS registrars and senior house officers in all departments of the hospital.

Although there is no doubt that this regular teaching commitment added greatly to the workload of medical staff it also required the support and understanding of nurses and the acceptance of some inconvenience by patients. Rarely were complaints made by any of these groups in the knowledge that being part of the teaching scene of a famous medical school brought prestige to the hospital.

Mention must also be made of in-service training for junior staff of the hospital and of educative exercises in general for all staff. The surgical unit for example started unit clinical meetings in 1951,[27] and the medical unit took a regular part in the presentation of cases and research material to the weekly meetings of medical units in the Edinburgh Northern Hospital group. At first, these meetings took place in each hospital in turn but were later centred at the Western General Hospital with its better meeting and presentation facilities. In 1968 a regular Thursday lunchtime meeting at which all units and departments of the hospital presented cases or papers was inaugurated.[28] These were intended initially for junior hospital staff and senior students but from the start local general practitioners were welcome and the importance of this component of the meeting increased over the years. These meetings continue, now with a wholly general practitioner purpose, with invited speakers and generously sponsored by drug firms.

The Role of the Hospital as an Examining Centre

Assessment of progress in knowledge and skills is an essential part of teaching and the acquisition by examination of degrees and diplomas is essential to the practice of medicine and the profession of a specialty. Leith Hospital in the last thirty years of its existence took an important part in these exercises. Clinical examinations in surgery for the final MB, ChB examinations of the University of Edinburgh took place at Leith and also clinicals in surgery and medicine for the finals of the Scottish Triple Qualification Examination (LRCPE, LRCSE and LRCPSG) from just after the second world war. Similarly examinations for the Fellowship of the Royal College of Surgeons of Edinburgh took place regularly and also for the Membership of the Royal College of Physicians of Edinburgh. Later the clinical examinations for the MRCP (UK) were conducted. This meant that the hospital was visited by many eminent surgeons and physicians from all over the United Kingdom as external examiners who were always delighted to return on similar occasions. For a short time clinical examinations in general medicine as part of the FRCS Edinburgh (Ophthalmology) were also conducted at Leith.

CHAPTER 8

REFERENCES

1. Leith Hospital Honorary Medical Staff Committee, Minutes 18.3.1896.
2. Ibid., 29.12.1898.
3. Ibid., 21.5.1908.
4. Marshall, J. S. (1986). *The Life and Times of Leith,* p. 114, Edinburgh; John Donald.
5. Leith Hospital Board of Managers, Minutes 21.4.1904.
6. Ibid., 9.2.1911.
7. Ibid., 10.5.1906.
8. Ibid., 21.3.1907.
9. Ibid., 13.3.1913.
10. Ibid., 18.10.1906.
11. Joint Committee on Post-Graduate Training, Minutes 20.12.1943.
12. Ibid., 3.1.1944.
13. Ibid., 14.2.1944.
14. Ibid., 6.3.1944.
15. Edinburgh Post-Graduate Board for Medicine, Minutes 7.5.1945.
16. Ibid., 6.6.1945.
17. Ibid., 10.12.1945.
18. Leith Hospital Honorary Medical Staff Committee, Minutes 14.12.1945.
19. Edinburgh Post-Graduate Board for Medicine, Minutes 10.12.1945.
20. Ibid., 26.12.1945.
21. *Chronicle,* Royal College of Physicians of Edinburgh (1975), Vol. 5, No. 3, p. 118.
22. Edinburgh Northern Hospital, Board of Management, Minutes 8.10.1957.
23. Ibid., 11.2.1964.
24. Ibid., 10.4.1964.

25.   Ibid., 17.10.1967.
26.   Ibid., 10.1969.
27.   Leith Hospital Clinical Staff Committee, Minutes 11.1.1951.
28.   Ibid., 28.5.1968.

CHAPTER 9

The Voluntary Support for the Hospital

The faithful financial support of innumerable citizens, rich and poor, of factories and ships and of bodies such as the Saturday Demonstration Committee and Hospital Fund Committee has already been recounted. Support for hospital activities can also be in the nature of services as well as on a monetary basis and Leith Hospital has been well served in this way. A number of organisations have contributed to the well-being of patients and staff and pre-eminent amongst these have been the Samaritan Society, whose function has already been alluded to briefly, the Women's Royal Voluntary Service, the Social and Fund Raising Committee and most recently the Ultrasound Machine Appeal.

Leith Hospital Samaritan Society
It is difficult for those brought up in the post Beveridge era to imagine the full consequences of lack of social welfare support on the sick during the last century and at the beginning of the present century. Sickness and poverty had a dire effect on each other, a circumstance unhappily still with us and highlighted so effectively by the Black Report on Inequalities in Health Care.

Effective continuing treatment and the ability to discharge patients from hospital were often frustrated by the patients' poor home and social conditions. There was as a consequence great scope for the Victorian and Edwardian propensity for charitable works. The need for such was evident to a particular degree in Leith which had seen some of the worst conditions in Scotland as the result of the industrial revolution. Fortunately the charitable instincts were strong and one result as far as hospital matters were concerned was the formation in 1908 of Leith Hospital Samaritan Society.

Its beginnings were modest. It began as an extension of the Leith Hospital Clothing Guild and at the first general meeting Mr Hutchison, honorary secretary of Leith Hospital explained that the work the society wished to undertake was the collection and distribution of clothing for patients leaving hospital or to purchase material and make it up. The lady members of the society were prominent members of Leith society and were often wives of local business and professional men. They elected Mrs Currie of Trinity Cottage as the Society's first president, Miss Ramage as vice president and Miss McNeill, honorary secretary and treasurer, and there was a committee of twenty-eight others. Their first year's income from subscriptions was £24.9.10.[1] Fund raising became an important part of the activities. Coffee mornings, sales of work, bridge parties and hospital balls all provided money and by 1984 money in bank accounts totalled £1,412 and money raised in that year amounted to £530.[2] The scope of their activities grew with the funds. Before the advent of the National Health Service they provided money for medical and surgical appliances for patients such as splints, callipers, artificial limbs and colostomy belts; clothing, food parcels and coal were given to the needy. They extended their work to areas regarded as amenities such as newspapers for the wards, a hospital library and Christmas parties for the children. Travelling expenses were provided for an entertainment party from the old Leith Alhambra Theatre.[3] The ladies provided cars for those going to convalescent homes and in particular a holiday scheme for children and "tired mothers" at Annsmill operated for many years.[4] In both world wars comforts were provided for members of the forces admitted to the hospital. These varied from warm underclothing to cigarettes, tobacco and handkerchiefs. Later the society provided money for some items of medical equipment. In 1926 a new operating table was provided for the children's wing[5] and into the 1980s during times of National Health Service financial stringency the medical staff had cause to be very thankful for equipment provided for them by the society.

It was clear that by the 1930s the committee was undertaking tasks carried out elsewhere by almoners and later by medical social workers. Individual cases were being discussed by name and visits made to homes before decisions to help were made.[6] Reference has already been made to the proposal put to the managers in 1933 that an almoner be appointed to the hospital, a decision being deferred however on receipt of a letter from the President of the Samaritan Society.[7] Nevertheless the ladies manifestly realised the limitations of their role as in 1934 they invited the almoner at Bruntsfield Women's Hospital to address them on "Almoner's Work".[8] Later when an almoner was appointed to Leith Hospital she attended by invitation meetings of the society and was frequently given sums of money to spend on her own initiative.

The redoubtable ladies of the Samaritan Society often saw their role as going beyond the welfare of poor patients and the provision of monies for hospital purposes. They were prepared to speak and act for the general good of the hospital. In 1937 the proprietors of the Eldorado dance hall, a close neighbour of the hospital, sought permission from the local magistrates to open an entrance to their hall opposite the hospital entrance. The committee sent a unanimous letter of protest against this unseemly request![9] Another example of practical aid was recorded at their meeting in February 1973 when a letter of thanks from the matron was read. It acknowledged the help given to the hospital during the one day auxiliary staff strike.[10]

One of the most imaginative and successful of the society's many enterprises was the inauguration in 1942 of the "Ship Ha'penny Fund" (these small halfpenny coins had a picture of a galleon in full sail on the reverse side). The fund provided for the endowment of cots for the children's wing and at least one was dedicated to the memory of all ranks of the British Mercantile Marine.[11]

They were also concerned in the 1940s about the position of the Society in relation to state owned hospitals. The local member of parliament, Mr James Hoy was contacted and in October 1947 the Society received a letter from him with the reassurance that on the takeover of hospitals by the state the Society would not be interfered with and would retain control of its funds.[12] This of course was true and it enabled the Society to continue to provide support to patients and hospital. The type of support inevitably changed. For example in 1955 it was decided to stop the outpatient parties for patients "as many of them greatly resented what they regarded as a charity gift!"[13] Nevertheless appropriate, generously given and very welcome service has been continued to the present time and will continue in whatever form the hospital exists in the future, the society in 1988 being led into these unknown waters by its president, Mrs Barbara Baker, secretary, Mrs Jill Davidson and treasurer, Mrs Daphne Green.

The Women's Royal Voluntary Service

There must be very few hospitals in the United Kingdom which do not benefit from the work of the ladies of this splendid organisation and gratitude is due to Mrs Wilkie MBE, regional organiser, Lothian WRVS for the following account of the service in Leith Hospital.

"WRVS has been involved in Leith Hospital for almost thirty years. It was in the early 1960s that WRVS was approached by the hospital management and asked if they could provide a shop/trolley service to the surgical and medical wards.

Initially there was opposition to the idea from the local shopkeepers, but when they were assured that we would not be undercutting their prices — WRVS shops etc. always sell at the recommended or "flashed" price — and that we would only be operating on one afternoon a week, they agreed to the scheme. We mainly sold soft drinks, toiletries, sweets, biscuits and writing materials and because we only operated once a week, stock was very limited. However, if patients desperately wanted something which we did not stock, the WRVS ladies were only too pleased to pop out to the nearest shop, and so a rapport was quickly established between the customers, the WRVS ladies and the local shop-keepers.

This system continued for about twenty years, until a greater demand for our service arose, principally because a lot of the smaller local shops had closed and patients and visitors found it easier to buy juice and other items from our trolley than carry them in from a distance. So we moved with the times, and volunteers were found to provide a ward trolley service on three afternoons, including Sundays.

Success breeds success and in 1984 the hospital suggested, not for the first time, that we should open a canteen/cafeteria for inpatients and outpatients, visitors and staff.

The hospital provided the facilities, the Eastern General Hospital (from the profits of WRVS projects there) provided the money to buy the essentials to start up and the local community responded magnificently to an appeal for volunteers to run it. The canteen opened in the spring of 1985, and has been much welcomed by patients and staff.

Now the old Leith Hospital is to be demolished to make room for a new one. We hope to have a part to play in this new hospital, but in the meantime, the WRVS ladies there have risen to a new challenge. WRVS are now the only providers of food in the premises, so with the addition of a microwave oven and a deep freeze to their existing facilities, they are now supplying sustenance to outpatients, staff and workmen.

From a handful of ladies working on their own in the sixties, we now have upwards of fifty volunteers working as a team in the hospital, for the benefit of the community, carrying on the tradition of service for which WRVS has always been known."

Leith Hospital Social and Fund Raising Committee

Despite the uncertainties and frustrations facing the hospital in the 1970s voluntary fund raising continued enthusiastically. The Social and Fund Raising Committee formed in 1978 had perhaps a wider base within and without the hospital compared to the Samaritan Society and in some respects was supplementary to that body.

Its main objective was to provide medical equipment which an increasingly constrained NHS was unable to do but it also provided gifts for patients. Its first chairman was Mrs Bainbridge, (Leith Hospital house steward), vice chairman Sister Fisher, secretary Mrs Brown, (medical secretary), and treasurer Mrs Downie, (receptionist/telephonist). One of its first efforts was the raising of £4,000 towards the cost of a patients' launderette in the geriatric assessment unit which had been proposed for the hospital, a proposal which was eventually dropped. The committee was then faced with the problem of how to use this sum, donated by the people of Leith for a specific purpose and it decided to help finance the restoration of the fire damaged "red court" which seemed inordinately delayed. Support from the clinical staff and the local management group was sought and obtained. On the initiative of Mr Roche, unit administrator, a meeting which included representatives of the Social Committee, Samaritan Society and medical and nursing staff was called and an attempt made to form a fund raising committee with a wide hospital and community base. Although it was stressed that this would be a "one-off" but major effort to provide funds for hospital development particularly with regard to the red court and which would be associated with the slogan "Raise the Roof for Leith Hospital", the individual components of the Steering

Committee did not gel. The committees and societies already in existence decided to continue their separate efforts and did so as enthusiastically as ever.

The Social and Fund Raising Committee, although it received some donations, raised most of its money by "street markets" each June. These took place in the old King Street car park of the hospital but also on occasions in the Rose Garden next to the outpatient department. All departments and organisations of the hospital took part by providing stalls selling baking, books, clothes, plants and even consultant surgeons and radiologists were to be seen expertly selling fish! Former patients were often in the midst of these activities. Gaiety was added to the day by Boys Brigade bugles and girls' marching bands and the opening was performed by a celebrity. These activities consistently raised between £1500-£2000 each year. The list of medical and surgical equipment provided is impressive and includes a colonoscope, retroscope, exhaled hydrogen monitor, cardiac recorders and many other items for the wards, physiotherapy department and casualty department. Some items as will be clear from the foregoing cost up to £5,000-£6,000.

The committee wound up its activities in 1986 but before doing so made the first substantial contribution of £1,000 to the Ultrasound Appeal Fund and many members contributed in a major way to the work of this appeal.[14]

Leith Hospital Ultrasound Machine Appeal Fund

This appeal with its outstanding success has to be seen as more than a mere money raising exercise. It was undoubtedly an expression of great affection for and loyalty to the hospital at a time when a threat of closure was in the air, shown by all members of staff, by patients past and present and by the community of Leith as a whole. The composition of the fund raising committee gives some idea of the wide support within the hospital. It included Sister Ferdi Fisher, children's theatre, Sister Julia Stewart, ward 4, Mrs Irene Downie, telephonist, Mrs Yvonne McClory, casualty receptionist, Miss Christine Lyon, paediatric secretary, Mrs Myra Mylchreest, administrative assistant, Miss Fiona Crawford, pharmacist, staff nurse Anne Watson, ward 4, Mr Iain Macintyre, consultant surgeon, Dr Douglas Grieve, consultant radiologist, Dr Michael Ford, consultant physician, Dr David Beamish, consultant anaesthetist, Mr Sinclair Bremner, superintendent radiographer and Mrs Lynn Lambie, physiotherapist who particularly devoted time and energy to the appeal. Essentially the sources of the funds raised were the people of Leith; pubs and clubs collected money in bottles and by raffles; there were street collections, sponsored walks and "bed pushes". A large raffle was run by the hospital and a grand auction sale took place in the Kirkgate Community Hall. The total amount raised was £36,000 of which £30,000 was needed for the machine, the balance being used for some other items of medical equipment.[15]

The machine itself is nowadays an essential piece of medical diagnostic equipment often replacing x-rays in the diagnosis of gall bladder, kidney and liver disease but at the time of the appeal patients at Leith Hospital had to be transferred to the Western General Hospital to have such investigations carried out. The benefits to patients in having the apparatus in the hospital were immense.

The ultrasound machine can be seen in the picture [plate 18] in which it is being handed over to Dr Douglas Grieve consultant radiologist by Dr D. Dunning, Chairman of Lothian Health Board and accompanied by Jim Calder, Scottish rugby internationalist, Hector Lambie, one of the sponsors, Russell Hunter, actor and Mr Iain Macintyre, consultant surgeon.

This then was the final expression of a community's involvement with its own general hospital before its demise.

CHAPTER 9

REFERENCES

1.   Leith Hospital Samaritan Society, Report 1908.
2.   Ibid., 1984.
3.   Ibid., 1920.
4.   Ibid., 1926.
5.   Ibid., 1926.
6.   Ibid., 1930.
7.   Leith Hospital Board of Management, Minutes 19.10.1933.
8.   Leith Hospital Samaritan Society, Report 1934.
9.   Leith Hospital Samaritan Society, Minutes 21.10.1937.
10.   Ibid., 22.2.1973.
11.   Ibid., 5.11.1942.
12.   Ibid., 10.10.1947.
13.   Ibid., 2.11.1955.
14.   Downie, Mrs Irene (1988). Personal Communication.
15.   Grieve, Dr D. (1988). Personal Communication.

Fight for Survival. 1971-1987

The community of Leith in the 1970s was vastly different from the community that had supported the opening of the hospital over a century before. The population had grown (at the beginning of the Second World War it was still around 80,000) but then waned as slum property was demolished and people moved elsewhere; industry and the port had thrived and then declined with the eventual loss of the ship building yards; and for a time after the war Leith was a somewhat depressed and depressing place. In the early 1970s however regeneration began to appear and much of it stemmed from a continuing sense of identity within the community. In 1972 the Port of Leith Housing Association was formed and dealt imaginatively with a major problem, and there is no doubt that the Scottish Development Agency in encouraging small industrial firms to establish themselves in special industrial sites and in supporting cleaning and refurbishing of buildings, helped greatly in the general increase in confidence.[1] Few citizens of Edinburgh would have considered any social activity in Leith of much attraction but recently a number of excellent restaurants, Asian and others, have been established in the port and to eat out in "Leith-sur-mer" has become socially acceptable!

Leith Hospital benefited from some of these activities such as stone cleaning of the building, but it is a pity that the general regeneration could not have extended to the overall function of the institution.

Changes in Administration

"I was to learn later in life that we tend to meet any new situation by reorganisation, and a wonderful method it can be for creating the illusion of progress while producing confusion, inefficiency and demoralisation." So said Caius Petronius of the Roman army in AD 66 and although many who experienced reorganisation of the National Health Service at first hand might see a parallel it would be harsh to suggest the effects were the same. Nevertheless the anticipation of and accommodation to reorganisation caused problems.

Leith Hospital's relation to the Board of Management of Edinburgh Northern Hospital Group and the South East Regional Hospital Board has been described. The Group Medical Superintendent, Dr Donald, retired in 1970 and was succeeded by Dr A. Anderson. Dr George Morris succeeded Dr Vaughan, with special responsibility for Leith Hospital, as deputy medical superintendent. Day to day matters at the hospital were supervised by him and by the matron with regard to nursing matters. Leith had never had an "on-site" administrator however until 1972 when Mr J. Roche was appointed as assistant administrator or hospital secretary. Before this, administrative staff at the Eastern General Hospital had had responsibilities for Leith. Regular supervision of the hospital fabric and function was also provided by the hospital "visitors", members of the Leith Hospital Committee who took it in turn, month by month in pairs, to inspect and report.[2]

Reorganisation of the National Health Service in 1974 saw the formation of the Lothian Health Board and the creation of North, South and West Lothian districts with Leith included in the North district. On 27th March 1974 the old Board of Management for Edinburgh Northern Hospitals held its last meeting at which appreciation was recorded of the work done by Councillor J. A. Crichton, a staunch supporter of the community of Leith, as the Board's last chairman. In turn, Mr Crichton said the Board could take credit for what had been achieved since 1948.[3]

The North Lothian District comprised hospitals of the old group namely the Western, Northern and Eastern General Hospitals and Leith but also Edenhall Hospital, Park House, Roodlands Hospital, Haddington, East Fortune Hospital, the Royal Victoria Hospital and Corstorphine Hospital. Dr J. B. P. Ferguson was appointed district medical officer with Dr R. C. S. Burnett, Dr H. D. Wilson and later Dr Armand-Smith community medicine specialists with some responsibilities for Leith. Mr A. L. Watt was appointed district administrator and Miss E. A. Edwards district nursing officer. As sector administrator, Mr K. Crichton had responsibility for Edenhall, Eastern General Hospital and Leith Hospital and Mr J. Roche who had been assistant hospital secretary was promoted unit administrator for Leith. Mr Roche was succeeded in 1980 by Mr J. Parry and subsequently by Ms Elizabeth Attenburgh, Ms Elizabeth Chubb and Ms Kathleen McKellar all of whom served as administrative assistants.

In less than a decade all hospitals were facing up to a further reorganisation with the introduction of general and unit managers. Leith had little time (or indeed enthusiasm) to appreciate and savour this further change which came into effect in 1986, a year before closure of inpatient facilities at the hospital. Dr Lindsey Burley was appointed general manager of the East Unit (comprising Leith, Eastern General Hospital, Edenhall Hospital, Roodlands Hospital and East Fortune Hospital). Mr K. Crichton became support services manager for the unit and Dr G. Venters community medicine specialist. Miss McKellar was the last administrative assistant to be centred at Leith. Dr Burley and her team, as will be described later, have the responsibility for implementing the future of services at Leith Hospital.

Work in a Hospital under threat of Closure

All aspects of Leith's activities in its last seventeen years as an acute hospital were coloured by a series of debates about its future. Uncertainties and delays with regard to firm decisions fed rumours with inevitable repercussions on staffing, improvement in services and morale. Nevertheless the hospital played an important part during this time in dealing with acute medical, surgical and paediatric emergencies from the Edinburgh area, in providing a service to local general practitioners and patients and in under-graduate and post-graduate teaching.

There was an overall reduction in inpatient and outpatient numbers seen particularly by 1986 (Table IX) when the dead-hand of closure was accepted. Other factors were operating however; some reduction of population around the hospital continued; the bed complement of the hospital fell again to 143 with closure of a surgical ward which was related to decreased need; the use of paediatric beds was particularly reduced with the opening of paediatric facilities in Fife and the final closure of the children's wing in October 1986;[4] the accident and emergency department had to limit its service; and finally with the free access to diagnostic facilities offered to general practitioners, fewer outpatient medical referrals were necessary.

The doubts about the viability of the accident and emergency department which had been expressed in the 1960s were voiced again in the 70s and 80s. The Scottish Home and Health Department recommended in 1981 that pre-registration house officers should not be employed in casualty departments which caused problems at Leith especially as they could not be adequately covered by more senior staff in the evenings and at weekends.[5] Attempts were made to maintain hours of opening but to limit workload but from 1983 it operated on a five day, 9 a.m. to 5 p.m., basis. It ceased work in 1987, Edinburgh thereby being left with two accident and emergency departments, one at Edinburgh Royal Infirmary and the other at the Western General Hospital.

The use of the medical wards during this time was made difficult (in common with all other acute medical units in the City) by the pressure on them during the winter and the difficulty in providing places for elderly patients requiring long term accommodation — the so-called "blocked bed" problem, which affected Leith particularly.[6] A discussion paper relating to the elderly in acute medical units produced by geriatricians in 1977 underlined this; a ward census in 1976 showed that 43 per cent of the bed complement was occupied by long stay patients (as compared to 15 per cent and 14 per cent for Eastern General Hospital and Western General Hospital respectively) and 72 per cent of admissions were sixty-five years or over. Leith also had one of the highest incidences of stroke admission in Edinburgh[7] and one of the highest incidences of "mandated" patients during the winter.[8] Mandated patients had to be accepted by medical units during periods of great demand for medical beds and as they tended to be elderly female patients living alone the accumulation of difficulties for an acute medical ward is apparent. Since the Lothian Health Board had an over-abundance of medical beds and an inadequate number of long-stay beds[9] solutions naturally presented themselves. These formed the basis of proposals that Leith medical unit be converted to long-term beds contained in a Lothian Health Board discussion paper of 1976.[10]

Despite all, the medical unit continued to function well. For example, although using the coronary care unit at the Western General Hospital appropriately, it was able to cope with the numbers of myocardial infarctions presenting to it with cardiac monitoring, defibrillating and emergency pacing facilities available. In 1980 a total of sixty-six patients with proven myocardial infarction (from 138 with chest pain) were admitted with a mortality in the under seventy age group of 5.8 per cent.[11] The medical wards continued to receive medical emergencies through the accident and emergency department and took its share of medical emergencies from the Edinburgh area. For many years also it increased its activity for several months during the winter by using the twenty beds in the empty surgical ward one to help with the general pressure on medical beds in Edinburgh at these times. This was done by engaging temporary nursing staff but with the existing medical staff.

The surgical unit continued its participation in the Edinburgh waiting day scheme and performed a wide variety of general surgical operations, with in its last full year an operative mortality of 0.3 per cent. Like the rest of the hospital however trends of activity in the last few years were downwards as can be seen from Table X.[12] The surgical unit played an important part in the provision of a gastrointestinal endoscopy service for the hospital. Contact with and involvement of general practitioners in the hospital was fostered during this time. They were welcome at weekly clinical meetings and annually from the mid 1970s a hospital staff/general practitioner evening was organised when problems of mutual concern were discussed and a buffet supper enjoyed on the hospital premises. Mention has been made of general practitioner access to hospital facilities. This was granted with regard to radiography in 1973,[13] physiotherapy in 1981[14] and electrocardiography in 1983. Upper gastrointestinal endoscopy had also been provided as an open access facility but had to be terminated in 1985 because of pressure on staff.[15] A further general practitioner link was forged in 1975 with the appointment of Dr A. R. Milne as a clinical assistant in the medical wards. Dr Milne took a particular interest in stroke patients in the wards, supervised outpatient diabetics and shared in the teaching of Phase III students.

One of the most disappointing of service losses in this time was that of post mortem examinations. From the early days autopsies were carried out in the hospital's own post-mortem room, after 1948 by pathologists from the department of pathology, Western General Hospital. By 1975 difficulties were being encountered because of poorly maintained facilities and lack of technicians.[16] Over the ensuing few years strenuous efforts were made to retain this important facility, but in the face of recommendations made in the Health and Safety at Work Act and the Howie Report (Code of practice for prevention of infection in laboratories and post-mortem rooms) and the fact that a figure of £40,000-50,000 was quoted as necessary to make Leith's post-mortem room satisfactory, no progress was made.[17] Clearly, the Lothian Health Board was unwilling to spend money for this purpose on a hospital whose future was in doubt and to the disappointment of clinical staff the South East Regional Committee for Post-graduate Medical Education refused to support retention of post-mortem facilities despite the implications for staff and student training.[18] From 1980 arrangements had to be made for the transfer of cadavers to the pathology department Western General Hospital which made the attendance of clinical staff at post-mortem examinations difficult or impossible.

There were however some areas of achievement and progress. The gastrointestinal endoscopy service was a very efficient one and was provided not only by surgeons but also physicians and in particular by Dr J. A. Forrest and Dr M. J. Ford. The activity of the x-ray department was maintained and increased with the introduction of an ultrasound service. Before 1980 this important service was available only at the Western General Hospital which did not provide a district service but was willing when possible to examine patients from Leith. This arrangement was often unsatisfactory and frustrating and led, as has been described, to a vigorous and successful fund raising campaign to provide a machine for Leith's own use on the premises.

It is even possible in the last decade of the general hospital to record an expansion of outpatient services. The psychiatric clinic started by Dr Lassalle in the 1960s had lapsed but in 1980 a clinic was restarted by Dr A. H. Jacques with the enthusiastic support of medical staff.[19] Dr Jacques also provided advice concerning psychogeriatric problems in the wards. In 1986, a drug dependency counselling clinic was established at Leith Hospital.[20] This coped with a significant number of local drug addicts but was run by staff from the City Hospital. A year later yet another service was started at Leith, by Dr George Bath, Community Medicine Specialist, Lothian Health Board. Housed in the outpatient department but again run by staff from without, the needle exchange service still operates in an attempt to reduce the spread of infection from the use of contaminated needles by drug addicts.

Although not part of the work of the hospital the local community nurses in the 1970s were granted accommodation in the basement of the main hospital from which to organise their invaluable domiciliary care. Later they also had some office accommodation in the nurses' home. The nurses' home it should be mentioned in passing changed its character and function in this time. Fewer and fewer nurses lived in and made use of the home and latterly post-graduate students were accom-

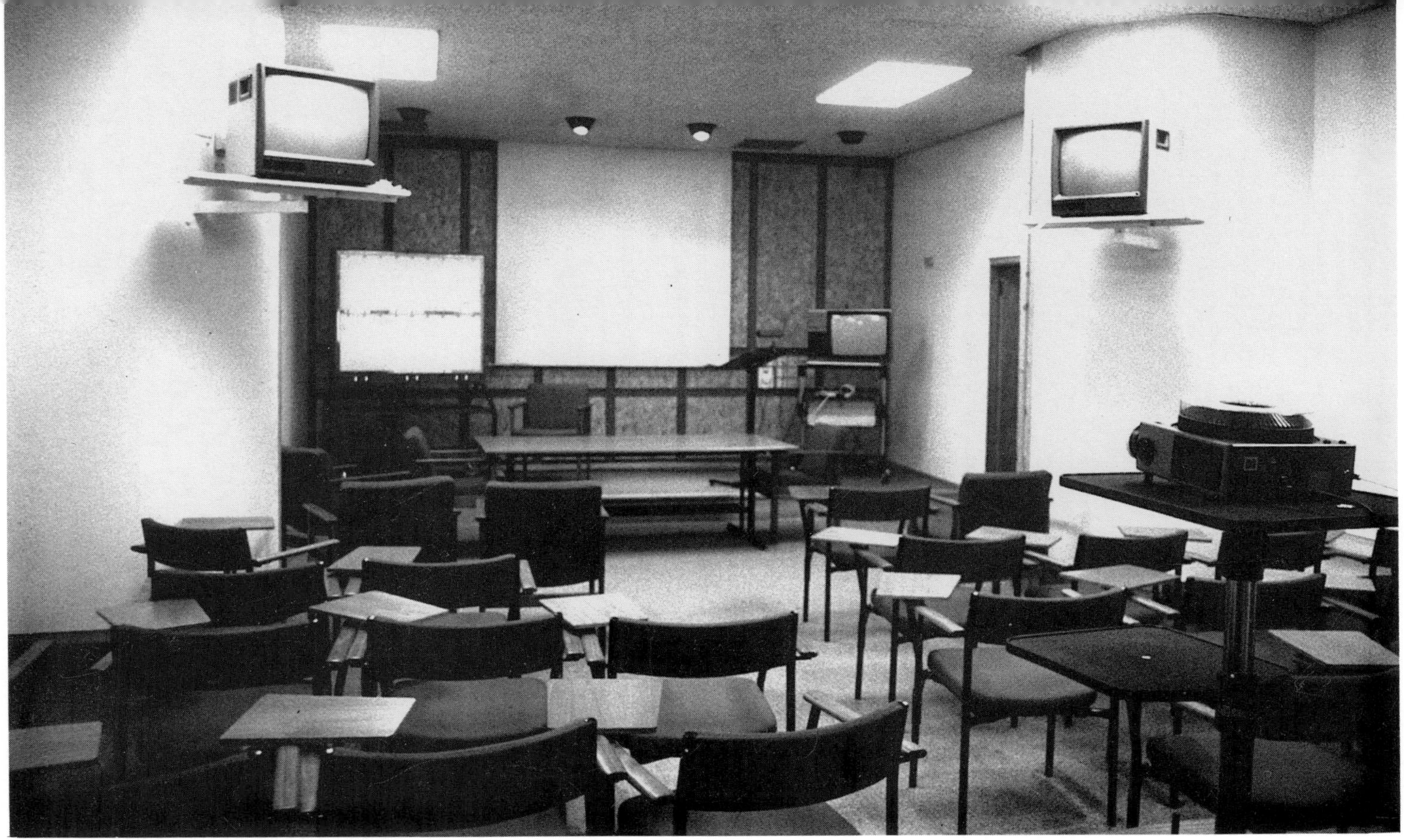

PLATE 21. The new conference room

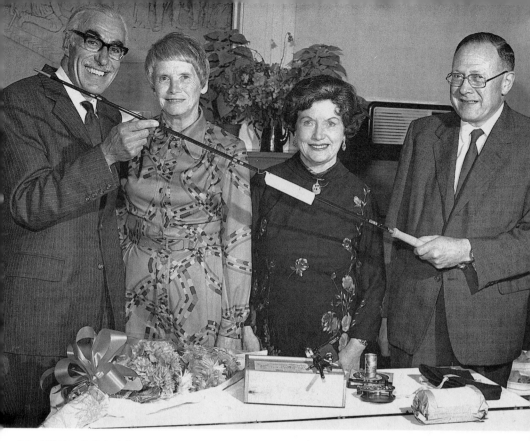

PLATE 22. Mr Eric Gilmour's retirement presentation, 1978. From left to right: Mr Gilmour, Mrs Gilm◦
Mrs Rena Nealon, Chairman of the Lothian Health Board and Dr R. F. Robertson, consultant physici◦

PLATE 23. Demonstration in support of the Accident and Emergency Department, 1983

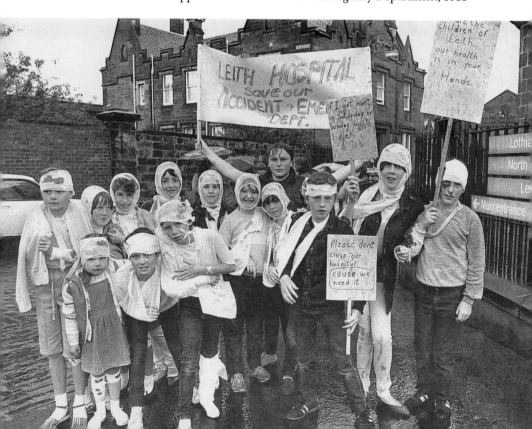

modated there adding some revenue to the hospital budget. The final sad chapter in the story of the home, not fifty years old, was the enforced closure in the 1980s because it failed to meet the standards of fire regulations.

The Work of Ancillary Departments in the Last Decade

Electrocardiography

In the 1950s the group medical superintendent was concerned with the pressure on the ECG service in the group and to avoid the need for the attendance of a technician at Leith Hospital and reduce the cost of transport, suggested the purchase of a direct writing machine for the hospital to be used by medical staff.[21] An ECG technician was appointed on a part-time basis in 1969 but she was based at the Eastern General Hospital attending Leith Hospital two days per week and did inpatient work only; in 1970 she carried out 590 ECGs. In 1973 Mrs Heggie the present technician was appointed and she attended Leith Hospital only, two hours per day on a daily basis, doing inpatient and outpatient work. In 1973, 690 tests were done and in 1986 2,336 patients (112 general practitioner) were seen. By that time however other inevestigations were added to simple ECG recordings. Exercise ECG's were started in 1974 and 24 hour ECG tapes in 1984. Mrs Heggie added simple pulmonary function tests to her repertoire in 1983.[22]

Radiology

Although a small three-roomed department with one part-time radiologist, a superintendent radiographer, Mr Sinclair Bremner, and three full-time radiographers and one clerkess, Leith Hospital x-ray department had 12,261 patient attendances in 1986 of which 890 were contrast examinations and 463 ultrasound examinations. From August 1987 it has served the outpatient clinics and general practitioners referrals only. The general practitioner access to this department has been maintained with full access to plain radiography, barium meal examinations, oral cholecystograms and intravenous urograms. There is also access to barium enemas and ultrasound after discussion with the radiologist, this being at pesent the only x-ray department in Edinburgh offering these procedures to general practitioners.[23]

Physiotherapy

Miss W. Ross, superintendent physiotherapist, supervised three full-time physiotherapists and one physiotherapist helper at Leith Hospital in 1986, a staffing level which was inadequate.[24] In that year 548 new inpatients and 1,061 new outpatients were seen which necessitated a total of 12,387 treatments. The usual physiotherapeutic problems were

K

tackled but particular efforts were made with regard to the rehabilitation of stroke patients and physiotherapists and occupational therapists frequently co-operated in making home assessments of patients due to be discharged in the struggle to maintain mobility and independence of elderly patients at home.[25]

Pharmacy

The pharmacy department at Leith Hospital was served with great devotion for many years by the pharmacist Miss Carruthers who on her retirement was replaced by Miss Coward. She was supported latterly by the unit pharmacist based at the Eastern General Hospital, Mr Prior.

Occupational Therapy, Speech Therapy and Medical Social Work

Leith Hospital did not have a full time member of any of these disciplines. Occupational therapists were shared with the Eastern General Hospital where the assessment unit was based and similarly a speech therapist (Mrs Dunlop) was shared. Mr John Goodey, medical social worker, had duties at the Western General Hospital as well as Leith. All three, however, were important components, with doctors, nurses, physiotherapists and chaplain (latterly the Rev. Gillian Morton) of the regular weekly "social round" when the inpatients social and family problems were tackled.

Medical Records Department, Secretaries and Chiropody

An efficient and cheerful group of workers performed the essential task of providing and retrieving hospital records. Many had served the hospital for long periods of time, the last medical records officer, Mr Rossbourgh, serving for a relatively short time. No clinician can function without the services of a good medical secretary and staff at Leith Hospital were particularly fortunate in this respect. For many years they were under the supervision of Mrs Allanach. A chiropody clinic operated within the hospital and a chiropodist attended inpatients on request.

Dietetics

Reference has been made to the limited dietetics service at Leith Hospital in the 1950s. In 1978 Miss Stoddart who had provided a dietetic service at the Eastern General Hospital and at Leith became district dietician for North Lothian. Thereafter a senior dietician based at the Eastern General Hospital provided an inpatient and outpatient service at Leith. At this time there was initiated a general practitioner referral service which expanded and when Lothian's first, and at that time only, community dietician was appointed in 1981 this general practitioner service was made her responsibility.

The most recent incumbent of the senior dietician post is Miss Fiona Steven and it is to her that gratitude is due for the following interesting digression on dietetics in the hospital. Provided with a copy of the minutes of the honorary medical staff committee for 12th June 1896, she was able to make interesting observations, comparing feeding practices then and now. The medical staff had, with the matron, met to consider the nutritional intake of both staff and patients. "There is no doubt," Miss Steven writes, "that food supplied to the patients was inadequate if they were only receiving half an ounce meat per patient at dinner. The main course portion sizes today would be between three and four ounces. One ounce of meat would supply only six grammes of protein and with a recommended daily amount of between sixty and eighty grammes per patient per day, they were obviously not going to achieve this from their meat intake, despite this being increased to one ounce similar to that given at the Royal Infirmary.

The practical suggestions given by the medical staff to vary the soups giving rice, lentil, pea, instead of just broth are amusing but undoubtedly of value. Their suggestion to increase the range of puddings to rice pudding, semolina, cornflour and tapioca along with saps are also beneficial. Insufficient variety in food intake is well accepted as a predisposing factor in malnutrition. As far as the quantity is concerned, it is difficult to assess the calorie content of the food supplied to the patients as there is insufficient detail about the total food provided to patients in Leith Hospital in 1896.

It is heartening that the medical staff and nursing staff recognised the importance of nutrition and its effect on the patient's prognosis. As a dietician working in the 1980s in the Health Service, I would say that I am still trying to make health care workers aware of the importance of nutrition.

The comments made on the staff meals are also interesting. Today, staff meals are decided by the Catering Manager in agreement with Unions. All staff should be ensured of having a wide variety of meals available but the staff are charged albeit at a subsidised rate. In the 1890s it would appear that this was obviously provided as part of the staffs' payment. It is little wonder they were unhappy about receiving breakfast at 6.30 a.m. and lunch at 1.45 p.m., with the morning being the hardest working part of the day. It is surprising that the variety of foods suggested included tripe, curry and Irish stew. Curry is perhaps the most popular item on our staff hospital menu.

I am grateful for the work done by Drs Stewart et al. They would appear to be pioneers of modern dietetics."

Miss Steven makes several other intriguing observations from other years. In 1904 the expenditure on food per patient per day was twopence; in 1987 the catering department's budget was £10 per patient per week! In 1944-49 there was no menu cycle, only seasonal fruits and vegetables were used, a cooked breakfast was given daily and chips were only rarely on the menu. In 1987 Leith Hospital had a three week menu cycle, a wide variety of fruits and vegetables were available as a mixture of frozen and fresh, a "continental breakfast" was provided for patients and the budget for fats and oils reflected the prevalence of frying. She finishes her comments by highlighting the difficulties facing the pharmacist in 1972 in producing a tube feed made up from Complan, glucose, Casilan, Prosparol and Orovite, compared with the ease of using present day commercially available feeds, and noting that in 1974 the dietician had to order five gluten free loaves per week from a local baker for inpatients on gluten free diets.[26]

Those who make other work possible

No-one with a knowledge of the work of a hospital can fail to appreciate the work of frequently unsung workers without whom any institution simply would not function. Leith has also been fortuante in these. A kitchen and catering staff under Mr Kelly, Unit Catering Officer, were all always anxious to demonstrate their skills for patients and staff. Engineers, under Mr Cormack, and tradesmen kept the fabric of the building in working order often under great difficulties of lack of money, and porters, latterly under Mr Harraughty, kept going essentially movement around the hospital at all times. Ward cleaners took as much pride in the appearances of the hospital as they did obviously in their own homes. All were part of a happy and efficient institution with the welfare of the patients their goal.

Alterations to Buildings — Successes and Failures

With the doubts about the future of the hospital ever present in the minds of planners and administrators it is not surprising that major extensions and improvements were eschewed. Nor is it surprising therefore that some parts of the hospital did not meet expectations of patients and staff in the 1980s. Improvements that were made tended to be piecemeal and as funds became available; patient toilets were improved and extended, day room facilities were improved and privacy, especially for ill, dying or noisy patients, provided in single cubicles. Improvement in decoration and the provision of oxygen supply, suction points and radio socketes to beds was continued. The old rather cold and institutional terrazzo floor of the Cowan Hall was covered with a fabric [plate 19] and a new much improved layout for the reception area in the hall was achieved. Some improvement in office accommodation in the x-ray department and for consultants was made but the doctors' dining room, for long a valuable meeting place for visiting staff and residents, was closed.[27]

In 1975 the North Lothian Division of Medicine recognised that each hospital should have an intensive care area or at least an intensive nursing area.[28] The medical staff had been unsuccessful in having a special care area provided in the 1960s but renewed their efforts in the late 70s and early 80s. The district medical officer requested that a paper be produced and this was done by Dr Mends, a community medicine specialist in a four page detailed report. The essential conclusion was that Leith Hospital had insufficient beds to warrant an intensive therapy unit but that an intensive nursing care section of four beds, linking two larger wards, might be viable but even this could only be supported "with some manipulation of the norms!"[29] It is perhaps not surprising that nothing further was achieved.

A development which occupied planners, administrators and clinicians for many man hours was the geriatric assessment unit. In the 1970s the Lothian Health Board's proposals on the redeployment of resources was discussed at length and as part of the exercise to increase the number of geriatric beds, a geriatric assessment unit was proposed for Leith Hospital[30] which was considered unsuitable for long term patients. Eventually, plans were produced and agreed in 1981[31] which envisaged the conversion of ward one and the offices and rooms on the north side of the old mortuary courtyard to such a use. To the disappointment of many this project was abandoned.

The most extensive rebuilding and reconstruction exercise carried out at the hospital in the last decade was forced on the authorities. In the morning of Sunday, 27th August 1978 a fire broke out in the hospital. It started in the Red Court area — the old Victorian Winter garden — and spread alarmingly, the initial flames having fractured an oxygen supply pipe. The last patients were being cleared from medical ward 7 by portering, nursing and medical staff as heat was cracking windows overlooking the court and some surgical patients had to be evacuated by a fire ladder from first floor wards. One elderly lady recovering from an operation told a reporter "We were chatting in the ward about 11.45 a.m. when the fire bell sounded. We all thought it was a practice but then smoke started to come in to the ward. It was terrible and we were all choking."[32] All sixty-eight patients helped to safety and a further twenty-two moved to the far end of one ward, praised all members of staff. Indeed the only worry that one lady had was that she was helped down a ladder by a fireman and was wearing only a short nightdress! The intensity of the blaze at its centre can be judged by the fact that coins in a nearby coin operated telephone were fused together. Fortunately there were no injuries but newspaper reports recorded £50,000 worth of damage.[33] From the first, the circumstances of the fire were suspicious and after police enquiries a man appeared in court on a charge of fire raising.[34] The badly damaged Red Court was essentially a communication space at ground level between surgical wards and the rest of the hopsital but fire damage was also done to the floor of ward seven and the old Board Room and it is not surprising therefore that a number of hospital services were temporarily crippled. The wider smoke damage was fairly rapidly put right but the temporary wooden corridors constructed through the Red Court in its roofless condition remained for several years. One of the difficulties facing builders and engineers was the fact that the courtyard, being at one time an external area, was laced with routes for drainage pipes, manholes and traps with a large heating mains to the surgical block.[35] The aspect of temporary wooden corridors in the middle of the hospital was a very depressing one but attempts to use endowment money to brighten the area were unsuccessful. It was not until 1984/85 that the availability of money made possible the reconstruction of the Red Court with extra offices, storage rooms, a WRVS canteen and shop and the creation of a new conference and teaching room. This added greatly to the amenity and function of the hospital but it is sad that it was to be enjoyed for so short a time. The appearance of the new Red Court and conference room can be seen in plates 20 and 21.

A temporary air of confidence was given to the hospital by these changes and also by the aforementioned external stone cleaning in 1985. Supported by the Scottish Development Agency, the facade of the children's wing and the north west end of the hospital including the entrance to the Cowan Hall and reception area were cleaned, revealing the original attractive colour of the sandstone.

Financial Matters in the Last Decade

Not a great deal can be said in this context with regard to a hospital not in control of its own financial affairs although some isolated facts may be of interest.

The hospital running costs for 1977-78 were £953,553. Of this, £685,874 went on wages and salaries, the major expenditure being on nursing salaries.[36] Running costs by 1985/86 had risen to £2,712,000 when the cost per inpatient week was £519.[37]

Money continued to be donated to the hospital and to be raised by various organisations described previously. Endowment funds were, of course, still operating. In 1980 North Lothian District Hospitals had as a general fund £16,024. Leith Hospital's general endowment fund held £37,961 with a further specific fund of £5,293. These funds provided for patients' comforts and Christmas festivities, for items of equipment, hospitality for guests, provision of television and radio and improvement to the main hospital entrance. There were however complaints about the use of endowment money in general. In 1981 the Edinburgh Health Council's sixth annual report recorded thirty-nine schemes taken off the Lothian Health Board's priority list for capital expenditure at a time of financial stringency but said that finance for such projects should come from the National Health Service and not hospital endowment funds. By 1986 general endowment funds were £109,385 and specific endowment funds were £27,995.[38]

Medical and Nursing Staffing

Dr D. H. A. Boyd was appointed physician to Leith Hospital, Deaconess Hospital and Longmore Hospital in September 1970. Following

Dr Chalmers Davidson's retirement and Dr Robertson's move to the Deaconess Hospital and Edinburgh Royal Infirmary in 1975 Dr Boyd had most of his sessions at Leith Hospital and some at the Western General Hospital. There followed a period of six years when five successive temporary or locum physicians shared the medical work with him. Those who stayed longest in these posts were E. B. French who retired in 1977, N. McD. Davidson who became physician to the Eastern General Hospital and Roodlands Hospital and J. A. Forrest who was appointed gastroenterologist to Stobhill Hospital, Glasgow. The reason for this very unsatisfactory state of affairs was the Lothian Health Board's indecision about the future of Leith Hospital and the discussions taking place concerning the creation of a chair of medicine based at the Western General Hospital.[39] The matter was not resolved despite representation by the North Lothian Division of Medicine to the Area Medical Committee, District Medical Officer and Chief Administrative Medical Officer[40] until 1981 when C. R. W. Edwards was appointed to the chair of clinical medicine at the Western General Hospital and P. L. Padfield as National Health Service consultant to the Western General Hospital and Leith Hospital. Professor Edwards also accepted responsibilities at Leith Hospital with the assistance of the Stanley Davidson lecturer, Dr Ian Hay, until both relinquished their duties at Leith in 1983. Professor Edwards with an international reputation in endocrinology, continues his teaching, research and service commitment at the Western General Hospital and Dr Padfield pursues his particular interest in hypertension also at the Western General Hospital. In 1983 Dr M. J. Ford was appointed to Leith Hospital and Deaconess Hospital. Ettles scholar of his year Dr Ford has a particular interest in gastrointestinal disease and did much to enhance the endoscopy service at the hospital. Now physician at the Eastern General Hospital he continues to run the medical outpatient clinic at Leith.

Mr Eric Gilmour retired in 1978, plate 22 recalling this occasion. He had been joined by Mr Graham Meikle in 1972, subsequent consultant surgical appointees being A. C. B. Dean, A. N. Smith, I. E. C. McIntyre, J. A. Saunders and I. F. MacLaren.

Graham Meikle, a second generation Rhodesian, was a meticulous general surgeon and examiner for the Royal College of Surgeons of Edinburgh; Allan Dean, a Senior Lecturer in the Department of Clinical Surgery was particularly interested in gastrointestinal surgery and was Chairman of the Examining Board of the RCSE; Adam Smith, a Reader in the Department of Surgery did most of his clinical work in the gastro-intestinal unit of the Western General Hospital and later became, very appropriately as regards the Leith appointment, Wade Professor in Surgical Studies in the RCSE.

Ian McIntyre had spent a period in a teaching post in South Africa and during his seven years at Leith worked endlessly to promote the well being of the hospital before leaving to become surgeon to the Western General Hospital. John Saunders, a Glasgow graduate, had a particular interest in gastrointenstinal endoscopy and had sessions at the Western General hospital. Ian MacLaren, surgeon to Edinburgh Royal Infirmary and Deaconess Hospital, returned to Edinburgh Royal Infirmary and continued his close ties with the Royal College of Surgeons of Edinbuirgh having been Secretary and Vice President.

Dr James Syme became full time paediatric physician at the Western General Hospital in 1984, further paediatric appointments during this time being Dr D. Barr, Dr Russell and Dr A. J. Burt who, appointed in 1984, still runs outpatient clinics. Mr Kirkland, paediatric surgeon, retired in 1985 but had been joined by Mr W. Scobie who still conducts outpatient clinics at Leith Hospital. Dr Loudon continued to conduct the gynaecology outpatient clinic until his retiral in 1987 and Dr Hughes maintained the ophthalmology outpatient clinic. Dr Beveridge relinquished the dermatology outpatient clinic in 1980 and was replaced by Dr J. A. Savin. After Dr Leslie Morrison's retirement in 1980, consultant anaesthetists were Dr E. Norman, Dr K. Dodd, Dr Janet Jenkins and Dr David Beamish who worked tirelessly in fund raising and hospital promoting activities. Dr Martin Fraser became full time radiologist for the Western General Hospital in 1978 and was succeeded by Dr Douglas Grieve who was another staunch supporter of the hospital and its activities in the last decade and still runs the x-ray department at Leith in addition to his other duties at the Western General Hospital.

In the 1970s the hospital functioned with seven house officers, three surgical, two medical and two paediatric. The surgical unit had an establishment of two registrars and one senior registrar and the medical unit one registrar and one senior house officer. The paediatric unit shared middle grade staff with the Western General Hospital. The medical senior house officer became part of hospital rotation schemes and also part of the South East Scotland vocational training scheme for general practitioners, both of which ensured incumbents of high quality.

Miss Bruce became senior nursing officer for Leith Hospital in 1975 and continued in this role until the closure of the hospital. She has however with her base at the Eastern General Hospital assumed responsibility for the nursing side of future planning at the hospital. She was aided in the last few years by a devoted group of senior nurses; Miss Wright, nursing officer and Sisters Loeb and Coutts night sisters; medical wards — Sister Forbes and Sister Brodie (with Sister Balfour as temporary Sister in the last few months); surgical wards — Sister Stewart and Sister Munro (with Sister Laidlaw temporary in the last months); paediatric wards — Sister Dickson (continuing as Sister in outpatient department) and Sister Muir; operating theatres — Sister Finlayson and Sister Couper; casualty department — Sister Irvine.

The Involvement of Community and Staff in the Hospital's Fate

The affection in which the hospital had been held by the community and the loyalty it had engendered in staff over the years must now be apparent. The reaction of Leith to the policies of the Health Board and the threat of closure may be therefore worthy of record.

Some services had been lost after the introduction of the National Health Service but more fundamental changes were being contemplated by the early 1970s and influenced for example, thoughts on the appointment of consultant staff.[41] [42] Conversion of medical beds to "second line" beds[43] was suggested as well as conversion or partial conversion to geriatric beds[44] but the North Lothian Division of Medicine backed away from these possibilities when contemplating the resulting pressure on other medical units.[45] Functional and staffing links both medical and surgical between Leith and the Western General Hospital were discussed.[46]

In December 1976 minds were very effectively concentrated by the publication of the Lothian Health Board's consultative document number one which suggested redeployment of acute hospital facilities and made clear that acute services were not thought appropriate for Leith Hospital. Redeployment, it was stated, however, did not mean closure of hospitals but changes in use.[47] Less than a year later consultative document number two was produced, the main proposals of this referring to Leith Hospital that it become a "Community Hospital" developed to meet the needs of the local population.[48] This implied retention of x-ray and physiotherapy services, outpatient clinics, two surgical wards, a non-major accident and emergency service and the upgrading of medical wards for geriatric patients. Consultative document number three on the long term development of hospital services made it clear that no acute inpatient services were contemplated for Leith Hospital.[49]

The response to these proposals was immediate and vigorous. Leith Community Association under the chairmanship of the Rev. Mrs Wardlaw totally disagreed with the Board's proposals and demanded that the entire surgical, medical and paediatric services be maintained.[50] Under the headline "All Parties Condemn Board Plans" a newspaper reported unprecedented condemnation by the four major political parties in Leith and Leith's member of parliament, Mr Ronald King-Murray, was quoted as being 100 per cent behind the people of Leith who wanted to maintain their local hospital.[51] Edinburgh District Health Council arranged a meeting which took place on 23rd February 1978 between local people and members and officials of the Lothian Health Board. This meeting is likely to pass into the legendary tales of Leith and its community; it was attended by over 300 people, chaired by Mrs Rina T. Nealon, chairman of the Board and proved to be a bruising one for many of its participants. There is no doubt that the intensity of local feeling was conveyed to the Board at this meeting and no doubt also that lay opinion was paralleled by medical views. The headline in the Leith Gazette "Consultants Fight on at Hospital" introduced an article in which among other points fears were expressed that the North Lothian District would have too few acute medical beds if Leith medical unit was closed.[52] By April of that year local campaigners were claiming victory in the battle to save the medical unit and were happy to have the issue in the hands of the Secretary of State. The Health Council in its report in 1978 described this as one of the major issues it had tackled and one of its greatest successes.[53]

Some idea of how opinion changed after 1978 can be gleaned from a memorandum on the implications of the Secretary of State's statement on the Health Boards future policy prepared by the district medical officer. In this document, improvements in the surgical wards, theatre, accident and emergency department and x-ray department were mentioned; a proposal that the children's wing be converted to a five day surgical paediatric ward was made and a proposal that a geriatric assessment unit be established was put forward. The bed complement for the hospital (apart from the twenty-bedded five day surgical paediatric unit) was proposed as surgical unit fifty, medical unit forty and geriatric assessment unit, thirty beds.[54]

So the hospital entered the 1980s but no sign of any of these proposals being implemented was evident. Disillusionment returned. In 1982 the medical staff invited Mr Ironside, chairman of the Lothian Health Board, to a meeting with them at the hospital when their concern with the delay and lack of overall planning of Leith Hospital's upgrading was expressed.[55] The following year a document — "Draft Strategy — A Framework for Development" was produced by the Lothian Health Board in which the 1970s policy of having no acute inpatient service at Leith Hospital was repeated. At the same time a feasibility study on alterations and extensions to Leith Hospital was made. A sum well in excess of two million pounds was said to be necessary[56] (the boilerhouse was on its last legs) and clearly no such amount was going to be spent on such old buildings (the oldest of acute hospitals in Edinburgh) unsuitable for upgrading to required standards. As previously indicated the accident and emergency department reduced its service in 1983 triggering another series of protests from the public. All sections of the community and all ages were involved and some protests as can be seen from plate 23 lacked nothing in dramatic content.

In May 1985 one newspaper article reflected a buoyant mood, suggesting that despondancy was disappearing and that Leith was a "hospital transformed". This was related to the external stone cleaning that had been done, the restoration of the Red Court area and the success of the ultrasound machine appeal.[57] A mere four months later the same newspaper bore a headline "Hospital Fears Resurface" and reported the view of Mr Ron Brown, Member of Parliament for Leith, that Leith could end up with a cleared site (of the hospital) that could be sold off to Barretts or Wimpey![58]

The final act began in October 1985 when yet another consultative document — "A Proposed Rationalisation of Hospital Services in North Edinburgh and Surrounds" was published by the Lothian Health Board. In it a timescale was given for the closure of the children's wing, the closure of surgical and medical units and the decomissioning of the hospital by September 1987. Once more opposition to the plans was voiced by the Edinburgh Health Council. A petition signed by 20 per cent of the population of the catchment area was handed in protest to a Health Board meeting. In December 1985 a meeting organised by Leith Community Association was held in the nurses' lounge in the hospital and voted 3-1 to reject the Health Board's plan for Leith Hospital. This time however the principle of the plan had been accepted by medical staff and one local general practitioner expressed the view that the hospital had met the needs of the 1940s, 1950s and 1960s but not the needs of the present time and certainly not the needs of the 1990s.[59] In September 1986 the Secretary of State approved the Board's proposals and the rundown to closure was started.

TABLE 9

Inpatient and Outpatient Statistics 1976 and 1986

	1976		1986	
	ADULT	PAEDIATRIC	ADULT	PAEDIATRIC
Inpatient				
Surgical	1454	725	843	415
Medical	743	571	713	188
Operations	?	?	919	?
(Endoscopies)			(454)	
Outpatients				
Surgical	1423	210	1198	155
Medical	409	154	554	118
Gynaecological	706		653	
Ophthalmic	409		249	
Dermatological	526		611	
Psychiatric			29	
Physiotherapy	1061		1610	
Counselling	—		75	
X-ray Department	8433*		6681	
E.C.G. Attendances	1311		2570	
Casualty Department	14013		5296	

* Adults and children

During the months that remained some members of staff retired, some found themselves posts elsewhere and others were transferred to other hospitals in the area. Clinical activity was gradually reduced with medical and surgical admissions ceasing on 26th June 1987 and the few remaining patients were transferred to appropriate care elsewhere by 31st July. Not in the 136 years of its activity had such stillness been experienced in the wards, corridors and departments. No whistling porters pushed patients between wards and x-ray departments; no anxious relatives walked with patients on their way to admission; no nurses chatted on change of duties; no students stood self consciously in new white coats; telephones were silent, food trolleys ceased their clatter. The resulting quietness was unnatural, disturbing and immensely sad.

CHAPTER 10

REFERENCES

1.   Marshall, J. S. (1986) *The Life and Times of Leith*, pp. 192-196, Edinburgh; John Donald.

2.   Edinburgh Northern Hospitals, Board of Management, Minutes 11.9.1956.

3.   Ibid., 27.3.1974.

4.   Leith Hospital Clinical Staff Committee, Minutes 19.1.1986.

5.   Ibid., 17.9.1981.

6.   Smith, R. G. and Lowther, C. P. (1974) *Blocked Beds — A Discussion Paper.*

7.   Lothian Health Board Statistics, 1975.

8.   Geriatrician Staff, Lothian Health Board, (1977). *The Elderly in Acute Medical Beds — A Discussion Paper.*

9.   *Scottish Health Statistics* 1982.

10.   *Lothian Health Board News (1976)*, No. 9.

11.   Fananapazier, L. (1980). Unpublished data.

12.   Leith Hospital General Surgical Unit, Saturday Morning Meeting, 21.2.1987.

13.   Edinburgh Northern Hospitals, Board of Management, Minutes 8.7.1973.

14.   Leith Hospital Clinical Staff Committee, Minutes 17.9.1981.

15.   Ibid., 25.7.1985.

16.   Ibid., 11.3.1975.

17.   Chairman of Leith Hospital Clinical Staff Committee Letter 22.11.1979.

18.   Secretary, South East Regional Committee for Post-Graduate Medical Education, letter 6.6.1980.

19.   Leith Hospital Clinical Staff Committee, Minutes 20.3.1980.

20.   Ibid., 19.1.1986.

21.   Edinburgh Northern Hospital, Board of Management, Minutes 11.11.1958.

22.   Heggie, Mrs (1987). Personal Communication.

23.   Grieve, Dr D., (1987) Personal Communication.

24.   Lothian Health Board (1986) Preliminary Report on Physiotherapy Services.

25.   Ross, Miss W. (1987). Personal Communication.

26.   Steven, Miss F. (1988). Personal Communication.
27.   Leith Hospital Clinical Staff Committee, Minutes 11.11.1975.
28.   North Lothian Division of Medicine. Report of Working Party to Consider Organisation of Hospital Care, 1975.
29.   Mends, Dr B. (1982). Intensive therapy in Leith Hospital: a report.
30.   Lothian Health Board (1979). Implication of the Secretary of State's statement on the Health Board's future policy — a paper.
31.   Leith Hospital Clinical Staff Committee, Minutes 10.12.1981.
32.   *Edinburgh Evening News*, 28.8.1978.
33.   *Leith Gazette*, 1.8.1978.
34.   Ibid., 8.9.1978.
35.   Letter from Senior Professional Officer, Common Services Agency, 18.2.1980.
36.   Leith Hospital Budget, 1977-78.
37.   Edinburgh Health Council Report 1986.
38.   Ibid., 1986.
39.   North Lothian District Division of Medicine, Minutes 30.7.1976.
40.   Ibid., 23.6.1978.
41.   Ibid., 28.6.1974.
42.   Ibid., 30.7.1976.
43.   Ibid., 25.3.1977.
44.   Ibid., 21.4.1977.
45.   Ibid., 21.4.1977.
46.   Ibid., 22.9.1978.
47.   *Lothian Health Board News* (1976), No. 9.
48.   Ibid., (1977), No. 11.
49.   Ibid., (1977), No. 12.
50.   *Leith Gazette* 20.1.1978.
51.   Ibid., 10.3.1978.
52.   Ibid., 23.12.1977.
53.   Ibid., 7.7.1978.
54.   North Lothian Division (1979), Report by District Medical Officer.
55.   Leith Hospital Clinical Staff Committee, Minutes 29.4.1982.
56.   Lothian Health Board Press Release, 14.7.1986.
57.   *Leith Gazette* 31.5.1985.
58.   Ibid., 13.9.1985.
59.   Ibid., 6.12.1985.

Epilogue. 1988 and Onwards

Although Leith Hospital has ceased to be as a general teaching hospital it will maintain a physical and functional presence in the community. The practical aspects of this transformation have been and will continue to be discussed at meetings of the Leith Hospital Development Group, which was set up at the end of 1986 shortly after the Secretary of State's decision on closure of the hospital. This Group includes Lothian Health Board staff, Leith Hospital staff, local general practitioners and representation from the Edinburgh Health Council. One of its earlier resolutions was that "The endowment fund would be continued to be used specifically by the present and the new Leith Hospital"[1] and one of its first acts was the setting up of a project team to consider details of organisation and building required. It accepted that one of its tasks would be to clear up misunderstanding in the community over the term "Community Hospital" and public expectations of this. Dr Venters as the Lothian Health Board community medicine specialist on the group has stated the Health Board's understanding of this, namely, the provision of sixty long stay beds, twelve general practitioner beds, a range of outpatient clinics and diagnostic and treatment facilities such as x-ray, physiotherapy and ECG.[2]

To achieve this, thought is being given to housing the outpatient clinics, to be run by visiting consultants, in a reconstructed children's wing, thus keeping what is Leith's 1914-18 war memorial with its recently cleaned exterior. The old outpatient building is likely to be used by community nursing staff. The Cowan Hall area, physiotherapy and x-ray departments will be kept and improved but the housing of the seventy-two beds is still to be decided. Present ward accommodation could be adapted or it could be demolished and rebuilt with new catering and heating units. To serve all this activity telephonists, receptionists, secretarial and medical records staff, tradesmen and auxiliaries will be required.

The Lothian Health Board has produced a brochure with the title "The New Leith Hospital". In it, future options are set out but some clear statements are made. The outpatient clinic services which are expected to be maintained are general medicine and surgery, paediatric medicine and surgery, gynaecology and ophthalmology, psychiatry, dermatology, special screening clinic and dietetics. The Board also mentions its consideration of bringing under one roof in the new hospital such community health service clinics as child health, dentistry, speech therapy, hearing testing, weight reduction and chiropody. It further expresses its wish to introduce outpatient clinics for obstetrics, orthopaedics, ENT and clinical psychology.

The final sentences of this brochure are, "The people of Leith have taken the present hospital to their hearts and given it support over the years. By responding with the same commitment to the opportunities provided by the new Leith Hospital the community can ensure that its needs are met in the same effective way as they have always been."

The commitment of the community of Leith seems assured. The commitment of the Lothian Health Board needs to be similarly assured. The people of Leith need to heed their own town's motto, "Persevere".

CHAPTER 11

REFERENCES

1.   Leith Hospital Development Group, Minutes 4.11.1986.
2.   Ibid., 11.3.1987.

APPENDIX I

Leith Hospital Senior Clinical Staff

Consulting Physicians	Appointed	Died
J. S. Combe	1851	1883
John Coldstream	1852	1863
James Struthers	1884	1891
John Henderson	1888	1901
G. W. Balfour	1892	1903
Claud Muirhead	1904	1910
Alexander Bruce	1904	1911
William Elder	1910	1931
H. G. Langwill	1912	1946
Edwin Matthew	1921	1950
H. L. Watson Wemyss	1931	1933
A. Murray Wood	1931	1945
G. D. Mathewson	1935	1936
T. R. R. Todd	1947	1975

Physicians, Consultant Physicians (NHS)	Appointed	Retired, Resigned, Died
William Elder	1897	1910
H. G. Langwill	1897	1912
John Eason	1910	1914
Edwin Matthew	1912	1921
A. Murray Wood	1914	1931
G. D. Mathewson	1921	1935
H. L. Watson Wemyss	1927	1930
T. R. R. Todd	1931	1947
G. L. Malcolm Smith	1931	1959
D. N. Nicolson	1936	1950
J. A. Bruce	1947	1950
R. M. Murray-Lyon	1948	1950
Chalmers H. Davidson	1950	1974
R. F. Robertson	1959	1975
D. H. A. Boyd	1970	1987

(Between 1975 and 1981 a number of temporary and locum physicians were appointed including S. R. Reuben, E. B. French, E. N. Wardle, N. McD. Davidson and J. A. Forrest.)

P. L. Padfield	1981	1983
C. R. W. Edwards	1981	1983
M. J. Ford	1983	

Consulting Surgeons	Appointed	Died
James Syme	1859	1870
James Spence	1871	1882
Sir P. Heron Watson	1883	1908
William Stewart	1906	1936
Alexander Miles	1913	1953
A. A. Scot-Skirving	1917	1928
J. W. Struthers	1925	1953
Sir David Wilkie	1925	1938

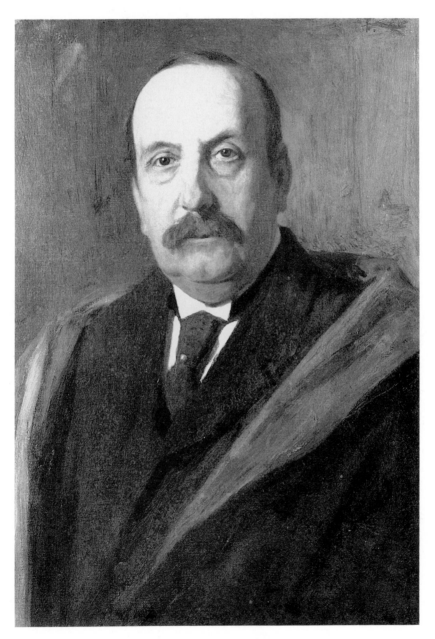

PLATE 24. Sir Patrick Heron Watson, 1832-1908

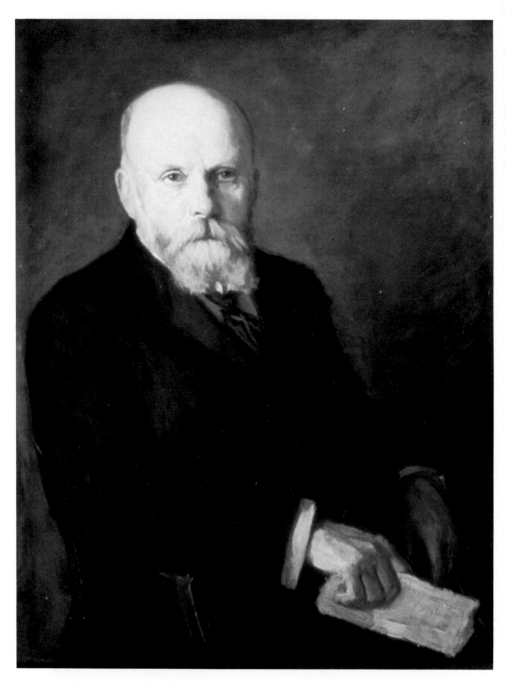

PLATE 25. Dr D. Berry Hart, 1851-1920

Sir Henry Wade	1927	1955
A. Pirie Watson	1938	1943
J. J. M. Shaw	1940	1940
J. R. Cameron	1967	

Consulting Urological Surgeon

David Band	1947	1988

Surgeons, Consultant Surgeons (NHS)	*Appointed*	*Retired, Resigned, Died*
William Stewart	1897	1906
Alexander Miles	1897	1910
A. A. Scot-Skirving	1906	1916
J. W. Struthers	1911	1925
Henry Wade	1920	1926
A. Pirie Watson	1925	1938
W. W. Carlow	1926	1950
J. J. M. Shaw	1927	1940
A. P. Mitchell	1938	1950
R. Leslie Stewart	1939	1944
David Band	1944	1947
J. R. Cameron	1947	1954
J. A. Ross	1947	1961
T. I. Wilson	1947	1966
Donald McIntosh	1948	1954
A. F. M. Barron	1947	1971
W. P. Small	1955	1962
I. E. W. Gilmour	1955	1978
A. I. S. McPherson	1962	1969
John Cook	1969	1972
Graham Meikle	1972	1980
A. C. B. Dean	1977	1981
A. N. Smith	1981	1984
I. M. C. McIntyre	1978	1985
J. H. Saunders	1981	
I. F. MacLaren	1985	1987

Consulting Gynaecologists	*Appointed*	*Died*
D. Berry Hart	1900	1920
J. Haig Ferguson	1911	1934
William Fordyce	1923	1941
W. F. T. Haultain	1933	1958
E. C. Fahmy	1947	1982

Gynaecologists and Consultant Gynaecologists (NHS)	*Appointed*	*Retired, Resigned, Died*
D. Berry Hart	1896	1900
N. T. Brewis	1900	1903
J. Haig Ferguson	1900	1911
William Fordyce	1911	1923
J. Lamond Lackie	1923	1925
W. F. T. Haultain	1925	1932
E. C. Fahmy	1932	1947
W. A. Liston	1947	1960

A. F. Anderson	1948	1959
J. D. O. Louden	1960	1987

Consulting Ophthalmic Surgeons	Appointed	Died
W. J. Sym	1906	1938
A. H. H. Sinclair	1912	1962
E. H. Cameron	1932	1983

Ophthalmologists and Consultant Ophthalmologists (NHS)	Appointed	Retired, Resigned, Died
W. J. Sym	1897	1906
A. H. H. Sinclair	1906	1912
H. H. Traquair	1912	1915
E. H. Cameron	1915	1917
E. H. Cameron	1921	1925
C. W. Graham	1925	1929
Laura M. Ligertwood	1929	1938
G. I. Scott	1938	1947
C. R. D. Leeds	1945	1965
G. S. Dhillon	1945	1964
J. Hughes	1964	

Dermatologists and Consultant Dermatologists (NHS)	Appointed	Retired, Resigned, Died
Robert Aitken	1931	1936
G. A. Grant Peterkin	1936	1971
G. W. Beveridge	1971	1980
J. A. Savin	1980	

Radiologists and Consultant Radiologists (NHS)	Appointed	Retired, Resigned, Died
Frederick Gardiner	1903	1906
F. R. Kerr	1906	1912
J. W. L. Spence	1918	1931
J. B. King	1931	1945
J. G. Kinninmonth	1937	1968
Martin Fraser	1968	1978
Douglas Grieve	1978	

Pathologists	Appointed	Retired, Resigned, Died
Theodore Shennan	1897	1903
W. T. Ritchie	1903	1907
J. D. Comrie	1907	1909
L. S. Milne	1909	1910
J. H. H. Pirrie	1910	1912
A. Pirie Watson	1912	1920
George Richardson	1920	1921
Andrew Rutherford	1923	1924
J. J. M. Shaw	1924	1925
R. Leslie Stewart	1925	1927
David Band	1927	1931
Bruce M. Dick	1931	1938

John Bruce	1938	1939
R. F. Ogilvie	1939	1948

Consulting ENT Surgeons	*Appointed*	*Died*
W. T. Gardiner	1929	1939
G. Ewart Martin	1937	1950

ENT Surgeons and Consultant ENT Surgeons (NHS)	*Appointed*	*Retired Resigned, Died*
J. S. Fraser	1912	1915
J. K. Milne Dickie	1915	1917
W. J. Gardiner	1920	1926
G. Ewart Martin	1926	1937
C. E. Scott	1937	1957
A. B. Smith	1945	1966*
J. F. Birrell	1948	1966*
J. R. McCallum	1952	1966*

*On transfer of unit to City Hospital

Anaesthetists and Consultant Anaesthetists (NHS)	*Appointed*	*Retired Resigned, Died*
H. Torrance Thomson*	1911	1924
Sybil Rutherford*	1928	1931
Miss D. A. D. Bannerman*	1931	?1945
Kenneth Herdman*	?1945	1955
L. G. Morrison	1955	1980
J. E. Norman	1964	1985
K. N. Dodd	1980	1985
David Beamish	1980	1987
Janet Jenkins	1985	1987

*General practitioners

Consultant Paediatric Physicians (NHS)	*Appointed*	*Retired, Resigned, Died*
D. N. Nicolson*	1948	1950
J. O. Forfar	1950	1964
A. J. Keay	1960	1970
J. Syme	1965	1984
D. G. D. Barr	1969	1974
Patricia Russell	1974	1985
A. J. Burt	1984	

*Previously appointed "physician".

Consultant Paediatric Surgeons (NHS)	*Appointed*	*Retired Resigned, Died*
F. H. Robarts*	1955	1965
Ian Kirkland	1955	1985
W. H. Bisset	1965	1971
W. G. Scobie	1971	

*Paediatric surgery previously undertaken by "surgeons"

APPENDIX II

Lady Superintendents and Matrons	Appointed	Retired, Resigned, Died
Miss C. M. E. Mackenzie	1874	1876
Miss Perry	1876	1892
Miss Paterson	1892	1908
Miss J. K. MacLean	1908	1929
Miss M. Wise	1929	1935
Miss M. W. Inglis	1935	1943
Miss A. M. McKee*	1943	1948
Miss McGregor Mitchell†	1948	1966
Miss J. H. Beale†	1966	1975
Miss S. N. Bruce‡	1975	

* Matron and deputy superintendent
†Matron
‡ Senior Nursing Officer

APPENDIX III

Presidents, Conveners and Chairmen, Board of Directors and and Managers	Appointed	Resigned, Died
William Stevenson, D.D.	1848	1856
Provost Taylor	1856	1860
Provost Lindsay	1860	1865
Mr Cochrane	1865	1866
Rev. Mr Thorburn	1866	1867
(Sir) William Miller	?1867	1886

(1887 — no president; vice-president, Charles Logan; Provost Aitken chaired.)
(1888 — no president; vice-president, Charles Logan; Baillie Archibald chaired.)

James Struthers	1889	1891
(Sir) John Struthers	1891	1897

(1898 no president; Mr Mitchell chaired.)

Very Rev. James Mitchell	1899	1910
Edmund Berry	1910	1922
Sir Richard Mackie	1922	1924
Ex-provost J. A. Lindsay	1924	1933
David Bell, J.P.	1933	1936
Sir Gilbert Archer	1936	1947
Captain W. D. T. Green	1947	1948

APPENDIX IV

Benefactors of the Hospital to 1941

1844	James Giles of Kailzie	£100
1851	John Stewart of Laverockbank, Leith	1,000
1851) 1853)	Alexander Cowan of Valleyfield, Penicuik	2,000
1853	Richard Grindlay, Leith	500
1858	John Ferguson of Carnbrock	100
1860	John Giles of Kinbyre	100
	Alexander White, Provost of Leith	1.000
	William Moodie, Leith	500
1863	Francis Lyon, Leith	500
1867	Mrs John Veitch, Leith	100
1868	Misses Elizabeth and Mary Sceales, Leith	200
	Mrs Marion Grandison	100
	Andrew Cowan, Leith	100
1872	Thomas Williamson Ramsay of Lixmount	24,855
	Miss Mary Wood, Hermitage Park, Leith	2,000
	Mrs Alexander Ferguson, London Row, Leith	200
1874	James Stocks, Newhaven Road, Leith	100
	Ebenezer Dewer, Wine Merchant, Leith	100
1875	Miss Aire, Leith	100
1877	Residuary Legatees of Mr and Mrs John Kay Wishart	300

1878   At the Annual Meeting of 1877, Mr James Wishart, Merchant, Leith, suggested that the Capital Fund should be raised to £20,000 by fifteen individuals giving £100 each. The suggestion was carried out by the following gentlemen. Mr Wishart heading the list:

	James Wishart, Leith	£100
	Stephen Adam	100
	J. Lindsay Bennet, London	100
	Robert Crawford, Leith	100
	W. J. Ford, Leith	100
	James Hay, Leith	100
	Provost Henderson, Leith	100
	John Livingston, Leith	100
	Graham Menzies, Edinburgh	100
	Robert Mowbray, Leith	100
	Sir William Miller, Bart, of Manderston	100
	Richard Raimes, Bonnington Park, Leith	100
	Peter Stocks, Leith	100
	James Struthers, M.D., Leith	100
	Robert Tod, Leith	100
	Peter Waddell, Leith 100	1,600
1879	Dr William Wood, R. N., London	504
1880	Peter McCraw, Leith	100
	Mrs Dewar, Bonnington Grove, Leith	100

1881   Miss Airth, the Founder of the Stead Benefaction, under whose Trust the Hospital receives two-thirds of the Revenue of a sum of £16,000.

	William Muir of Inistrynich	2,000
	Mrs Pirrie, Leith	200
1882	Henry Johnston, Stationer, Leith	130

1883	Muir Crawford, Merchants, Leith	100
1884	Capt. Alexander Blackwood, Shipowner, Leith	200
	Richard Raimes, Bonnington Park, Leith	200
1885	Mrs Elizabeth Hardie, London	500
1888	Mrs Ann White, Leith	100
	Mrs Sebastian Duncan, Leith	500
	James Wishart, Leith	250
	Miss Elizabeth Waddell, Leith	8,000
	Representatives of the late Richard Raimes	100
1889	Robert Tweedale, 45 Madeira Street, Leith	500
1890	James Taylor of Starley Hall	2,000
1891	Dr James Struthers, Leith, share of the Residue of his Estate	8,000
1892	John Crabbie, Leith	500
	William Milne, Hotel keeper, Edinburgh	200
1893	Richard Raimes, jun., Bonnington Park, Leith	100
	Miss Agnes Stocks, Newhaven Road, Leith	1,000
1894	William Gillespie, Lansdowne Crescent, Edinburgh	250
	Miss Millburgh Mowbray, Northumberland Street, Edinburgh	2,649
1895	Mrs Mackenzie, 9 Middle Arthur Place, Edinburgh, bequest of Property in Queen Street, Leith, which realised	257
1896	The Earl of Moray	2,500
	Peter Waddell, Claremont Park, Leith, one-fourth share of the Residue of his Estate, estimated at	25,000
	James Watt, The Falcons, Leith	1,000
1897	To Endow a Bed in memory of the late Mr Geo. Dobson, Timber Merchant, Leith — from one of his Beneficiaries	1,600
	Miss Jessie Robb, Ferry Road, Leith, one-third of the Residue of her Estate	1,211
	Miss E. G. Mowbray, Northumberland Street, Edinburgh	100
1898	Robert Slimon of Whitburgh	1,000
	To Endow a Bed "In grateful acknowledgement of services rendered to a Trust by William Thomson, Esq., Shipowner; Christian Salvesen, Esq., Shipowner; and Thomas Aitken, Esq., Merchant, all in Leith	1,600
1899	Mrs Laughton, 1 Park Road, Trinity	100
	Subscribers to the Leith Commemoration Scheme of the Queen's Diamond Jubilee, with accrued interest	4,986
1900	Mrs Agnes Mackenzie, 55 Cleveland Square, Hyde Park, London	100
1901	Dr John Henderson, Leith	1,000
	Thomas K. Hardie, Esq., London, the interest whereof is desired by the testator to be applied towards carrying out the objects of the Hospital	1,000
1903	To Endow a Bed from "One of Ourselves"	1,600
	To Endow a Bed from "Another of Ourselves"	1,600
	To Endow a Bed to be called "Samaritan Bed," from Miss Cant, 8 John's Place, Leith	1,600
	Scottish Co-operative Wholesale Society, Limited	250
1904	Mrs Jessie Reid, Rosemount, Ferry Road, Leith	450
1906	Mrs Elizabeth Murphy, West Newport, Fife	500
1907	To Endow a Bed from John Jordan	1,500
	William Thomson, Esq., and James Wishart Thomson, Esq., to Endow a Bed in Leith Hospital in memory of their father William Thomson, Esq., of Craigbinning, Shipowner, Leith	1,500
	An Anonymous Donor	1,000
	A friend, per James Ross, Esq., 8 James Place, Leith, being a special	

donation (with interest) to the Capital Funds of the Hospital 1,015

1908   James Wishart Thomson, Leith 500

Hugo Knoblauch, Leith 500

Thomas Aitken of Nivingston 1,000

John S. Gibb, 31 East Claremont Street, Edinburgh 500

A. & R. Tod, Ltd., Leith 500

Mrs Joan Paxton, 62 Fountainhall Road, Edinburgh 100

John Warrack, Esq., Shipowner, Leith, for endowment of beds 50

1909   To Endow a Bed in memory of their Father, the late James Ford,
from James Johnston Ford, 16 Rothesay Terrace, Edinburgh,
£750; and Patrick Johnston Ford, 8 Moray Place, Edinburgh, £750 1,500

Miss Bridget Mary Davison, Boswall House, Boswall Road, Leith 500

James Wilkie Dunlop, 6 Gloucester Crescent, Regent Park, London 250

Miss Margaret Rennie M'Nair, 2 Summerside Place, Leith 200

Various amounts received towards endowment of beds 140

1910   Trustees of David Sim White, Bonnington, Edinburgh 1,000

Anonymous Donation to Endow a Bed in memory of King Edward
VII 1,500

Anonymous 500

Trustees of Charles Anderson, of Fettykill 1,000

Miss Mary Hardie Mungall, 12 Queen's Crescent, Edinburgh 196

Peter Thonson, of Binny 180

Captain William Reid, 12 Craighall Crescent, Leith 100

1911   William Johnston Ford, Merchant, Leith 4,000

Anonymous, to Endow a Bed to be named "Coronation" 1,500

Trustees of Charles Anderson, of Fettykil 1,546

Mrs Muir, Madeira Street, Leith 100

Donations received for Mr John Hislop's Children's Cot Scheme 1,016

1912   John Thomas Donaldson, 189 Newhaven Road, Leith 100

Trustees of Charles Anderson, of Fettykil 1,000

Trustees of David Jamie, Edinburgh 1,000

Miss Elizabeth M'Laren, 43 Summerside Place, Leith 100

William Thomson, Shipowner, Leith 450

Miss Annie Chapman Douglas, Forthside, Lennox Row, Trinity 770

Anonymous Donation to Endow a Bed to be named "Miss Elder" 1,500

The Very Reverend James Mitchell, D. D., sometime Minister of
South Leith Parish Church, legacy to Endow a Bed 1,500

1913   Peter Whyte, C.E., 4 Magdala Crescent, Edinburgh, to Endow a
Bed to be called "The Leith Docks Bed" 1,500

1913   The Widow and Children of the late James Wishart Thomson, to
Endow a Bed in his memory 1,500

Martin Julius Ellingsen, Merchant, Leith 500

1914   Robert Lindsay, Curator, Royal Botanic Gardens, Edinburgh,
share of residue 897

Rev. Dr Struthers, balance of residue 457

1915   Legacy from John Jordan, Merchant, Leith 2,000

Miss A. C. Douglas, residue of estate 556

Legacy from John Campbell, 45 Summerside Place, Leith 100

One-fifth residue of said John Campbell's estate 304

Mrs Galloway, 9 Bellevue Crescent, Edinburgh, to Endow a Bed
in memory of her husband, M. P. Galloway, Shipowner,
Leith 1,500

Mrs Grant, 3 Manor Place, Edinburgh, to Endow a Bed in memory
of her nephew, Lieut. Mungo Campbell Gibson, R.N. 1,500

Gretna Memorial Fund to Endow a Bed and Cot in memory of the

Officers and men of the 1/7th Royal Scots who lost their lives in the Gretna Railway Disaster 2,487

1916 Legacy from Captain D. A. Lindsay, 5th Royal Scots 100

Col. and Mrs Lyell, Redfern, Colinton Road, Edinburgh, to Endow a Bed in memory of their son, Lieut. David Lyell, 7th Royal Scots 1,500

Mrs Campbell Gibson, 7 Buckingham Terrace, Edinburgh, to Endow a Bed in memory of her husband, Campbell Gibson, Shipowner, Leith 1,500

Anonymous 10,000

Mrs Kennedy, 15 Palmerston Place, Edinburgh, to Endow a Bed in memory of her husband, Frederick Charles Kennedy, C.I.E. 1,500

1917 Legacy — Mrs Elizabeth Hunter, 114 M'Donald Road, Edinburgh 100

Legacy — Owen Hughes, retired Stevedore, 7 Charlotte Street, Leith 100

Trustees of late Charles Anderson, of Fettykill 624

1918 Miss Helen M. Inglis, 47 Murrayfield Gardens, to Endow a Bed in memory of her brother, Thomas Inglis of Glenternie and Woodhouse, Peeblesshire 1,500

Mrs Thomson and the Misses Sarah Wishart Thomson and Barbara Louise Thomson, Glenpark, Balerno, Midlothian, to Endow a Bed in memory of 2nd Lieut. Kenneth Douglas Thomson, Argyle and Sutherland Highlanders 1,750

Mrs Garland, 53 Charlotte Street, Leith, share of residue 1,071

1919 Mrs Jessie Campbell, Currie, Trinity Cottage, Trinity — Legacy of Cottage Convalescent Home, Corstorphine, with all furniture and Equipment.

Mrs Jessie Campbell Currie's Sons and Daughters, towards maintenance of Convalescent Home 5,000

John Storrie, 17 Wester Coates Avenue, Edinburgh — Legacy 100

1920 (National War Bonds). In memory of the late Mr Thomas D. Dobson, Timber Merchant, Leith, from one of his beneficiaries 2,000

1921 Trustees of the late Miss Dawson, of Gairdoch and Powfoulis 375

Legacy from Francis Moffat Haldane, Ellerdale, Moffat 200

The Misses Ford, Avenel, Colinton Road, Edinburgh, to Endow Bed in Female Medical Ward in memory of their parents, the late Mr Thomas Ford and Mrs Jane H. C. Ford 2,000

Thomas Cowan, 10 Henderland Road, Edinburgh, Shipowner, Bed Endowment, £5 per cent. War Stock, 1929-1947 5,000

Mr Cowan, on behalf of a Friend of the Hospital, to cover cost of Electric Motor 200

Residue — William Lyall's Trust 108

1922 Mrs R. E. Harvey, 24 Drumsheugh Gardens, Edinburgh 102

Trustees of the late Miss Dawson, of Gairdoch and Powfoulis 1,200

Anonymous 500

Thomas Cowan, Shipowner, 10 Henderland Road, Edinburgh 5,000

Trustees of the late Andrew Richardson, retired Examining Officer, H.M. Customs, Leith, half share of residue 921

Trustees of the late John Inglis, of Woodhouse Manor, Peeblesshire 1,750

1923 Trustees of the late Miss Dawson, of Gairdoch and Powfowlis 800

Legacy from John Wilson, 23 Royal Terrace, Edinburgh 200

Residue — James Mackay's Trust 150

Legacy from Mrs Janet Guthrie Robson, Lauder 315

Thomas Cowan, 125 Constitution Street, Leith 10,000

Voluntary Hospitals Commission 1,010

1924   Trustees of the late Miss Dawson, of Gairdoch and Powfoulis 1,000
Legacy from Janet Burns or Taylor, 11 Chamberlain Road, Edinburgh 100
Voluntary Hospitals Commission 1,060
James Mackinlay, 87-89 Constitution Street, to Endow a Bed in
     memory of his late father.. 1,750
Trustees of Peter Macdougal, Victoria Mount, Lennox Row, Trinity,
     to Endow a Bed in memory of Misses Christian and Margaret
     Macdougal, and the said Peter Macdougal... 2,080
Trustees of James G. Bridges, of Merleton, Boswall Road, to Endow Beds .. 5,625
1925   Mrs Paterson, 20 Murrayfield Avenue, for the purpose of providing
     X-Ray Installation as a memorial for her late Husband, Dr Wil-
     liam Paterson, Leith 1,000
Trustees of the late Miss Dawson, of Gairdoch and Powfoulis 500
British Charities' Association (Grant) 165
1925   Thomas Cowan, Shipowner.. 500
Trustees of James G. Bridges, of Merleton, Boswall Road, addi-
     tional to Endow Beds 1,500
Misses Sarah Wishart Thomson and Barbara Louise Thomson,
     Glenpark, Balerno, to Endow a Bed in memory of their late
     mother, Mrs Barbara Grey Thomson.. 1,750
David S. Crawford, Bellevue Bakery, to Endow Cots 1,000
1926   Mrs Corsar, Belmont, Murrayfield, cost of Cots 445
Seven-a-side Rugby Football Tournament... 250
Trustees of Miss Dinah M. Dawson, of Gairdoch and Powfoulis.................... 700
Trustees of the late John Wilson Bequest Fund 150
Legacy from Mrs Elizabeth Salter or Murphy, Newport, Fife (additional) 500
Thomas Cowan, Shipowner... 500
Legacy from Charles John Woodard, 89 Willowbrae Avenue, Edinburgh 100
Trustees of James G. Bridges, of Merleton, Boswall Road, addi-
     tional, to Endow Beds 600
1927   Thomas Cowan, 10 Henderland Road, Edinburgh 500
Mrs A. J. Ferguson, 28 Palmerston Place, Edinburgh (Proceeds of
     Leith Hospital Ball) 143
Trustees of the late Miss Dawson, of Gairdoch and Powfoulis 700
Trustees of the late John Wilson Bequest Fund 200
Eleven Grandchildren of the late Mrs Joan Galloway, 9 Bellevue
     Crescent, Edinburgh, in loving memory of their
     Grandmother.. 550
Trustees of the late James Stewart Dunbar, of Langshaw, Dumfriesshire........ 250
Miss Annie Collie Miller, 88 Duke Street, share of Residue........................... 221
Seven-a-side Rugby Tournament 250
Miss Annie Nicolson Hunter; Mrs Margaret Hume M'Neill; Mrs
     Joy Forrest; John Galloway Galloway; Matthew Percy Galloway;
     Alfred Douglas Galloway; Bruce Stirling Galloway, to Endow a
     Bed in loving memory of their mother, Mrs Joan Galloway, 9
     Bellevue Crescent, Edinburgh.. 1,500
"Leith War Memorial" Committee Endowment Purposes 26,222
1928   William Tulloch, Merchant, 10 Hermitage Place, Leith.............................. 4,587
Thomas Cowan, Shipowner, Leith 500
Andrew Cunningham, Craigend, Ferry Road, Leith (Balance of Legacy)........ 450
Mrs A. J. Ferguson, 28 Palmerston Place (proceedings of Leith Hospital Ball) 250
Seven-a-side Rugby Tournament 300
Trustees of Miss Dawson, of Gairdoch and Powfoulis 600
Trustees of John Wilson Bequest Fund 300
Mrs Jane Rutherford, 15 Annfield, Newhaven.. 100

1928	Leith Provident Co-operative Society, Ltd., to Endow a Bed	1,750
	William Crawford & Sons, Ltd., Biscuit Manufacturers, Edinburgh, to Endow a Bed in memory of the late Mr William Crawford	1,750
	Trustees of James G. Bridges of Merleton, Boswall Road, to Endow Beds. Balance of Legacy	1,443
	To Endow a Bed in memory of Mr and Mrs Christian Salvesen, from their sons and daughters	1,750
	Anonymous to Endow the "Earl Haig" Cot	1,500
	Mrs A. C. Murdoch, St Kilda, York Road, Trinity, to Endow the "Annie C. Murdoch" Cot	1,000
1929	Thomas Cowan, Shipowner, Leith	500
	Mrs A. J. Ferguson, Firrhill, Colinton (proceeds of Leith Hospital Ball)	275
	Trustees of Miss Dawson of Gairdoch and Powfoulis	600
	Trustees of John Wilson Bequest Fund	500
1929	Mrs Mary Kennedy Carlekemp, North Berwick	150
	Legacy from Sir James Wishart Thomson, K.B.E., Shipowner, Leith	2,500
	One much interested in Leith Hospital and its work — for Radium	100
	Mrs J. Abernethy of Bush, Milton Bridge — for Radium	100
	Seven-a-side Rugby Football Tournament	262
1930	East of Scotland Football Association (Rosebery Charity Committee)	170
	Thomas Cowan, Esq., LL.D., 10 Henderland Road, Edinburgh	500
	Trustees of late Miss Dinah M. Dawson of Gairdoch and Powfoulis	550
	Mrs A. J. Ferguson, Firrhill, Colinton (Proceeds of Leith Hospital Ball)	409
	Seven-a-side Rugby Football Tournament	210
	Trustees of John Wilson Bequest Fund	300
	John Warrrack, Esq., Shipowner, Leith, for Endowment of Beds	50
	Donations received for Mr John Hislop's Children's Cot Scheme	1,016
	Various amounts received towards Endowment of Beds	140
	Trustees of Edward Clark, Printer, Edinburgh	2,000
	Trustees of Miss J. B. Mackie, Zurich	300
	Trustees of Mrs J. S. Hall, Tweed Villa, 130 Newhaven Road	100
	Trustees of Joseph Darling, Millburn Cottage, Torphichen.	100
	Trustees of Archibald Darling, Millburn Cottage, Torphichen	4,008
	Trustees of Miss Christina Laing, 5 Gladstone Place	5,750
1931	Thos. Cowan, LL.D., 10 Henderland Road, Edinburgh	500
	Edinburgh and Leith Wholesale Wine & Spirit Trade Association	100
	Trustees of Miss Dawson of Gairdoch and Powfoulis	450
	East of Scotland Football Assoc. (Rosebery Charity Committee)	176
	Trustees of John Wilson Bequest Fund	150
	Two Sisters	100
	Leith Provident Co-op. Society Employees' Charity Organisation	110
	Edward Clark, Printer, Edinburgh, per his Trustees	1,000
	Miss Catherine Jane Wilson, 26 Woodville Terrace, Leith, per her Trustees	100
	Arch. Darling (deceased), Millburn Cottages, Torphichen	3,014
	David Robertson, Chalmers, 15 Grange Terrace, Edinburgh (of Messrs D. Robertson & Son, Elbe Street, Leith), per his Executrix, Miss C. C. Chalmers	2,000
	Wm. Walker, Shipowner, Leith, per his Trustees	1,680
	Mrs A. J. Ferguson, Firrhill, Colinton (Proceeds of Leith Hospital Ball)	420
1932	An Old Leither — An Ex-Patient	100
	Trustees of Miss Dawson of Gairdoch and Powfoulis	250
	East of Scotland Football Association (Rosebery Charity Committee)	100
	Mrs A. J. Ferguson, Firrhill, Colinton (Proceeds of Leith Hospital Ball and Bridge Party)	434
	Seven-a-side Rugby Football Tournament	167

Trustees of John Wilson Bequest Fund 150
The late D. M. Gammie, 15 Mayfield Gardens 481
The late Alex. Lillicoe, St Dunstane Villa, Melrose 250
Trustees of the late Edward Clark, Printer, Edinburgh 500
The late Mr and Mrs Robert Montgomery, 41 Liberton Brae, Edinburgh 1,400
1933   Trustees of the late Mr David Davidson, Stationer, 9 Bernard Street, Leith.. 3,300
Trustees of the late Mr David Ferguson, Merchant, Leith 28,000
Mrs Mary Kennedy's Trust to Endow a Bed to be named the "Mary
    Kennedy" Bed 2,000
Trustees of the late Mr William Sharp, 17 Glenorchy Terrace, Edinburgh 1,000
The late Miss Mary Gordon Scott Wallace, 2 East Fettes Avenue,
    (per Miss C. C. Chalmers) 500
1933   Trustees of Miss Dinah M. Dawson, of Gairdoch and Powfoulis 250
Trustees of the late Mr Andrew Aikman, Constitution Street, Leith 280
Executrix of the late Miss Janet Archibald, 1 Restalrig Terrace 181
Trustees of the late Mr John Wilson, Merchant, Edinburgh 150
Mrs A. J. Ferguson, Firrhill, Colinton (Proceeds of Leith Hospital Ball) 441
Murrayfield Seven-a-side Rugby Football Tournament 165
East of Scotland Football Assoc. (Rosebery Charity Committee) 100
Leith Provident Co-op. Society (Proceeds of Joint Co-op Exhibi-
    tion, Dalmeny Street Hall) 223
Edinburgh, Leith and District Pleasant Sunday Evening, Leith Branch 100
1934   Trustees of the late Edward Clark, Printer, Edinburgh 500
Trustees of the late David S. Crawford, Edinburgh 5,000
Trustees of the late Mrs Anna D. A. Chetham, 4 Bowhill Terrace, Edinburgh 100
Trustees of the late Mrs Agnes Deans, 3 Largo Place 100
Mrs Ferguson, Firrhill, Colinton, Proceeds of Bridge Party and Ball
    for "Sunshine Verandah" (Children's Wing) 453
Trustees of the late David Ferguson, Constitution Street (Eye
    Department) 10,000
Mrs Salvesen, 21 Buckingham Terrace, to Endow a Bed by the late
    Mr F. G. Salvesen in memory of his five nephews who died in the
    War 1914-18 2,000
Scottish Hospital Fund (Duke of Atholl) for Capital Expenditure purposes ... 400
Trustees of the late Miss Dinah M. Dawson, of Gairdoch and Powfoulis 225
Edinburgh, Leith and District Pleasant Sunday Evening (Leith Branch) 100
Seven-a-side Tournament, Murrayfield 150
Trustees of the late John Wilson, Merchant, Edinburgh 100
1935   Trustees of the late Mrs Jessie Black, 123 Dudley Avenue, Leith 610
Proceeds from the Bridge Party and Ball, organised by Mrs
    Haultain and Mrs Alex. Ferguson (for Sunshine Verandah) 310
Miss Campbell M. Currie, Trinity Cottage (for Cottage Home) 200
Trustees of the late Miss Dinah M. Dawson, of Gairdoch and Powfoulis 175
The Leith Churches' Wireless Fund 163
Seven-a-side Rugby Football Tournament, Murrayfield 160
Trustees of the late Mr Alexander Mackie, 4 Laverockbank Terrace,
    Trinity (for Children's Wing) 100
Trustees of the late Mr John Wilson, Merchant, Edinburgh 100
East of Scotland Football Assoc. (Rosebery Charity Committee) 100
1936   Trustees of the late David Ferguson, Esq., Constitution Street, Leith
    (Residue) 5,790
Trustees of the late Thos. Cowan, Esq., LL.D., 10 Henderland
    Road, Edinburgh 2,500
R. W. Cuthill, Esq., Edinburgh, to Endow two Cots in Children's
    Wing in memory of Bobbie Costa 1,000

Trustees of the late Mrs M. J. Munro, Inverbervie, Craighall Road, Leith 500

Mr and Mrs Jas. Reid, 3 Craighall Gardens, to Endow Cot in Children's Wing in memory of their son, James William Reid 500

Trustees of the late Mrs Eliz. Still, 313 Easter Road, Leith 355

Trustees of the late Miss R. C. Warrack, 5 St Margaret's Road, Edinburgh 300

Proceeds from Bridge Party and Ball, organised by Mrs Haultain and Mrs Alec. Ferguson, for Building Appeal Fund 295

East of Scotland Football Assoc. (Rosebery Charity Committee) 250

1936   Trustees of the late Sir Malcolm Smith, K.B.E., Clifton Lodge, Boswall Road, Leith 200

Seven-a-side Rugby Football Tournament, Murrayfield 160

Trustees of the late Miss Dinah M. Dawson of Gairdoch and Powfoulis 150

Trustees of the late Mr John Wilson, Merchant, Edinburgh 100

1937   Trustees of the late James Cormack, Esq., Shipowner, Leith 6,000

Trustees of the late Miss J. R. Tod, 67 Ferry Road, Leith 5,122

Trustees of the late Wm. Prentice, Esq., 21 N. Junction Street, Leith 679

Trustees of the late Alex. Campbell Cormack, Esq., Shipowner, Leith 500

Trustees of the late James Cormack, Senr., Shipowner, Leith 459

Proceeds from Bridge Party and Ball, organised by Mrs Haultain and Mrs Alec. Ferguson 173

"A Samaritan" 200

Trustees of the late Miss Dinah M. Dawson of Gairdoch and Powfoulis 175

East of Scotland Football Assoc. (Rosebery Charity Committee) 150

In memory of Robert William Cuthill Costa (1910-1935) 100

Trustees of the late Samuel Brown, Esq., 34 Dock Street, Leith 100

Trustees of the late Hugh Mears, 18 Buchanan Street 100

Trustees of the late Mr John Wilson, Merchant, Leith 100

Seven-a-side Rugby Football Tournament, Murrayfield 100

1938   The late Miss M. O. Taylor, to Endow a Bed, "Thomas and Margaret Burns Bed" 2,000

Ralph Nicholson, Esq., Chancelot Cottage, to Endow a Cot in memory of Ralph Henderson Nicholson 500

Trustees of the late Miss Dinah M. Dawson of Gairdoch and Powfoulis 250

Bridge Party and Ball, per Mrs Haultain 220

Murrayfield Seven-a-side Tournament 145

The late Mr Wm. Prentice 118

Heart of Midlothian Football Club 112

The late Mrs Euphemia Mackenzie, 4 Ruskin Terrace, Great Western Road, Glasgow 102

The late Miss Jessie Chisholm, 27 Cambridge Gardens, Leith 100

The late Mrs Mary Pinkard, 38 Saughton Crescent, Edinburgh 100

In memory of Robert William Cuthill Costa (1910-1935) 100

The League of Mercy 100

1939   Hospital Ball, per Mrs Haultain — Of which £50 to the Building Appeal Fund 250

Murrayfield Seven-a-side Tournament 150

Trustees of the late Miss Dinah M. Dawson of Gairdoch and Powfoulis 225

Trustees of the late Mr John Wilson 250

Anonymous 784

The late Mr John Cochrane, 44 Kirkgate, Leith 100

The late Miss Mary Fraser, 68 Comiston Drive 2,000

The late Miss H. S. Grant, 13 Park Road, Leith 100

The late Mrs Charlotte D. Mill, 14 Glencairn Crescent 500

The late Mr Thomas Reekie, 118 Newhaven Road 450

The late Mr Donald Henderson Dunbar, 15 Stanley Road, to

Endow a Bed, the "Dunbar Bed" 1,350

The late James Currie, Esq., LL.D., Shipowner, Leith, Cottage
Home Endowment 1,000

1940 Trustees of the late Miss Dinah M. Dawson of Gairdoch and Powfoulis 200

Trustees of the late John Wilson 250

The late Mrs Georgina M'Niven, 48 Brunstane Road 3,500

The late Miss C. C. Chalmers, 15 Grange Terrace 1,000

1941 The late Mrs Georgina McNiven, 48 Brunstane Road, further on account ...1,754

The late R. C. Mouat.. 453

The late Miss A. A. White, 23 Glencairn Crescent....................................... 500

The late Miss Agnes McIntosh, 1a Summerside Place.................................. 100

Trustees of the late David S. Crawford...1,000

The late Mrs Campbell Gibson 200

The late Wm. Leslie, 28 Cornhill Terrace 666

The late Wm. Thomson, Shipowner...1,000

The late Miss Cath. B. Grier, 10 Rosslyn Crescent...................................... 500

The late Miss C. C. Chalmers, 15 Grange Terrace 781

A Shipmaster's Widow and Daughter — Two Cots to
commemorate "The gallant Scottish Merchant Servicemen of all
grades" 1,000

The late T. Douglas Dobson, Timber Merchant, to endow two beds,
"Douglas and Agnes Dobson Beds"... 5,000

The Trustees of the late Miss Dinah M. Dawson, of Gairdoch and Powfoulis.. 200

John Wilson Bequest Fund 250

Henry Robb Ltd. 150

Cinematographers Exhibitors' Association 100

Index

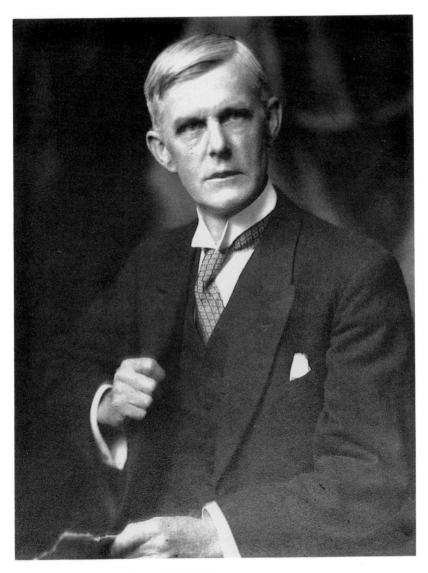

PLATE 26. Sir Henry Wade, 1877-1955